PRAISE FOR

ISA CHANDRA MOSKOWITZ & TERRY HOPE ROMERO

VEGAN CUPCAKES TAKE OVER THE WORLD

"[Moskowitz and Romero] produce insanely fetching cupcakes with mousse fillings, butter cream frostings, chocolate ganache icings and sprinkles galore."
—*New York Times*

❖

"Packed with 75 dairy-free recipes and lush photos aimed at making vegans and omnivores drool." —*Washington Post*

❖

"Written chattily and supportively for even the most oven-phobic ... reading this is like having a couple of fun, socially conscious post-punk pals over for a slumber party ... Each page of this cookbook contains an irresistible delight."
—*Bust*

❖

"Work your way up from amateur to vegan cupcake master of the universe."
—*VegNews*

VEGANOMICON

"The very same urban chefs who had you inhaling vegan butter-cream frosting
during your free time have crafted the next revolution in neo-vegan cuisine."
—*Philadelphia City Paper*

❖

"[Moskowitz and Romero] are as crude and funny when kibbitzing as they are subtle and
intuitive when putting together vegan dishes that are full of non-soggy adult tastes."
—*New York Times Book Review*

❖

"Exuberant and unapologetic... recipes don't skimp on fat or flavor,
and the eclectic collection of dishes is a testament to the authors'
sincere love of cooking and culinary exploration."
—*Saveur*

❖

"The *Betty Crocker's Cookbook* of the vegan world." —*Bitch*

VEGAN COOKIES

INVADE YOUR COOKIE JAR

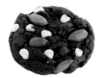

ALSO BY

ISA CHANDRA MOSKOWITZ & TERRY HOPE ROMERO

Veganomicon

Vegan Cupcakes Take Over the World

ALSO BY

ISA CHANDRA MOSKOWITZ

Vegan Brunch

Vegan with a Vengeance

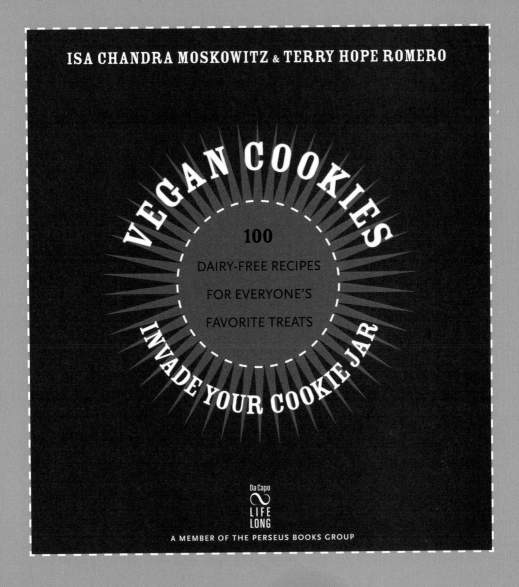

ISA CHANDRA MOSKOWITZ & TERRY HOPE ROMERO

VEGAN COOKIES

100

DAIRY-FREE RECIPES

FOR EVERYONE'S

FAVORITE TREATS

INVADE YOUR COOKIE JAR

Da Capo
∞
LIFE
LONG

A MEMBER OF THE PERSEUS BOOKS GROUP

To the memory of Bea Arthur, we know you're eating vegan cookies in heaven.

Many of the designations used by manufacturers and sellers to
distinguish their products are claimed as trademarks. Where those designations
appear in this book and Da Capo Press was aware of a trademark claim,
the designations have been printed in initial capital letters.

Text and photography copyright © 2009 by Isa Chandra Moskowitz and Terry Hope Romero

Editorial production by *Marra*thon Production Services, www.marrathon.net
Adapted from original design by Pauline Neuwirth, Neuwirth & Associates, Inc.
Set in 10.5 point Whitman

Cataloging-in-Publication data for this book is available from the Library of Congress.

ISBN 978-1-60094-048-4

Published by Da Capo Press
A Member of the Perseus Books Group
www.dacapopress.com

Da Capo Press books are available at special discounts for bulk
purchases in the U.S. by corporations, institutions, and other organizations.
For more information, please contact the Special Markets Department at the Perseus
Books Group, 2300 Chestnut Street, Suite 200, Philadelphia, PA, 19103, or call
(800) 810-4145, ext. 5000, or e-mail special.markets@perseusbooks.com.

First Da Capo Press edition 2009

10 9 8 7 6 5 4 3

CONTENTS

INTRODUCTION

COOKIES NEED no introduction.[1] They're cookies. Unless someone has been working in the chocolate chip factory all day and they just can't stand the sight of them, when you offer a cookie the answer will almost always be "Yes." Or maybe an "I really shouldn't ..." while they reach for one, anyway.

They are the perfect casual treat. After all, who wants to greet their new neighbors with a tray of tiramisu or welcome their child home from school with cherries jubilee? And you certainly can't send that chocolate mousse pie via mail. Just the very phrase "a plate of cookies" tugs at our heartstrings like a basketful of wide-eyed puppies.

As soon as we were able to preheat the oven, we were baking cookies. They are an excellent introduction to the world of baking. Minimal equipment is needed and the ingredients list is usually succinct and to the point. Get the whole gang together and dropping, rolling, or shaping cookies becomes effortless and fun. Cookie baking time is blessedly short; some can even be out the door with you in half an hour if an emergency bake sale is taking place in the town square. Indeed, baking cookies is a necessary skill for any superhero, no cape required.

In this book we've brought together about

---

[1] They *need* no introduction, but we're giving them one anyway.

100 of our favorite cookie recipes. From classic favorites like OATMEAL RAISIN COOKIES (page 75) and our version of the New York bakery staple, NYC BLACK AND WHITE COOKIES (page 161), to new inventions like FROSTED GRAPEFRUIT ICEBOX COOKIES (page 201) and GREEN TEA WALNUT BISCOTTI (page 209), we've taken to our test kitchens with wands and crystal balls to create cookie magic. We won't sleep until we've veganized the world! Or maybe we just enjoy wearing the big floppy wizard hats.

Our love of cookies ... all kinds of cookies ... has driven our relentless quest to find a sweet little treat for most every moment or situation in your life. Homemade veganizations of familiar cookies will have those childhood hankerings covered, whether it's a peanut butter sandwich cookie or a big fat crispy rice square. No gluten? No problem—we have substitution solutions for all. You believe that cookies should be part of a well-balanced diet? So do we! A selection of wholesome cookies that makes use of minimally processed sweeteners and whole grains will keep you feeling pristine. And of course, if there's a cookie season to celebrate it's

those winter holidays. You'll find plenty of gorgeous, crazy-festive recipes that will make you the life of the cookie swap. From sparkling sugar cookies for the kids and Irish cream liqueur–reminiscent frosted whiskey cookies for the grown-ups, no unsuspecting cookie nosher would imagine that it's all vegan, and any vegan will know that this is the way cookies were meant to be. There is no such thing anymore as "real (not vegan) cookies" when great vegan cookies look and taste this delicious.

So perhaps that unhappy person who said "food is not love" has never had a cookie. The simple act of breaking apart a chocolate chip cookie, still warm from the oven, is an iconic tableau of the American childhood experience. Whether you had that experience yourself as a child, or desperately need to compensate in your adult life, we're here for you. Vegan cookies *are* invading your cookie jar. Don't run and hide, there's no escaping it. It's sweet, sweet surrender!

With love from Portland and Queens,
   Isa Chandra Moskowitz and
   Terry Hope Romero

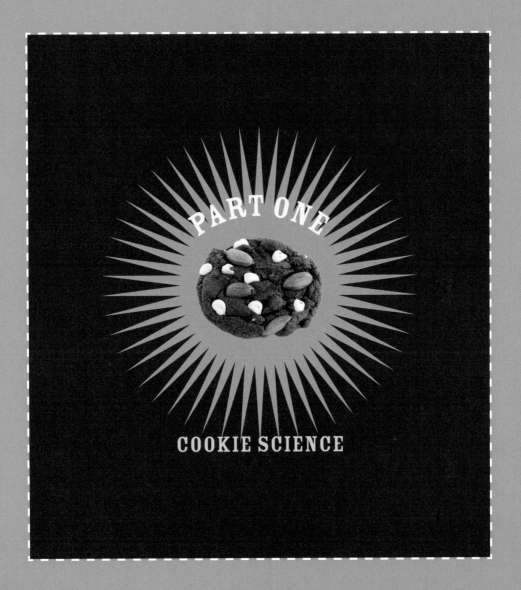

PART ONE

COOKIE SCIENCE

INGREDIENTS
Make 'Em Your Best

YOUR COOKIES are only going to be as good as your ingredients. Well, eating most any cookie is better than eating a scoop of flour, but you get our meaning—investing in quality flours, pure flavor extracts, and the best chocolate chips, fruits, and nuts you can get your hands on is key for taking your cookies from "Hey, good cookie" to "Will you spend the rest of your life with me?"

Many of the following ingredients may already exist in your pantry. If you plan on serious baking, it's always a good idea to take stock ... it's no fun to run out of rolled oats or brown sugar mid–oatmeal cookie mixing! Even if you're planning on only making one particular recipe, it doesn't hurt to have plenty of the "extras" on hand, just in case inspiration strikes and you suddenly need to make chocolate-oatmeal-macadamia-sesame-raspberry jam cookies.

You can make your cookies as organic as you please. Organic ingredients (flour, sugar, extracts, etc.) function the same as their nonorganic counterparts in these recipes.

Use the following ingredient list to guide your next shopping trip if your pantry is looking bare. We've listed items in the order of largest to least volume in a recipe; you'll need several cups of flour and just a little bit of baking soda, for example.

IMPORTANT FLOUR MEASURING TIP ALERT
THE MISMEASURE OF MAN

For accuracy, we always use the "scoop-and-scrape" method of flour measuring. It's also useful for measuring cocoa powder and other dry ingredients. Simply use your measuring cup to generously scoop up some flour, enough so that the cup is overflowing. Gently tap the side of your cup; this helps the flour settle and eliminates any tiny air pockets. Finally, use the back of a knife to scrape the excess flour from the top of the measuring cup to create an even, flat surface. Flour to the people!

FLOURS

The "bones" of a cookie start with a good flour. Most of the cookie recipes in this book call for old reliable all-purpose, but don't let anything stop you from replacing up to half the amount with whole wheat pastry or whole wheat white flour—you'll get more fiber with excellent results. See our substitution guide (page 27) and check out the Wholesome Cookies chapter (page 93) if you'd like to experiment even further with healthier baking.

ALL-PURPOSE FLOUR is the most commonly used, thanks to its accessibility, consistent results, and neutral flavor. It's made from wheat that's had the dark germ and bran removed. Sometime it's further whitened by bleaching but we don't go there ... look for unbleached all-purpose flour with its characteristic off-white hue.

WHOLE WHEAT PASTRY FLOUR: All of the nutrition of whole wheat flour, but light and delicate, too? Sign us up. Whole wheat pastry flour is a baker's dream and it's typically organic as well. This delicate flour is ground from wheat berry that naturally has a lower gluten content. It will give your whole-grain baked goods a lighter texture and flavor than if you used regular whole wheat flour. It's interchangeable with all-purpose flour, so you can switch in half of a recipe's all-purpose flour content with whole wheat pastry to increase the fiber and nutrition without upping the characteristic grainy "health food" flavor. But if you're feeling super-whole wheaty, go ahead and use all whole wheat pastry—crazier things have been done.

WHOLE WHEAT WHITE FLOUR: Whenever a new kind of whole wheat flour hits the supermarket shelves we sit up and listen, and with whole wheat white flour we like what we're hearing. Whole wheat white is ground from hard white wheat berries; it's lighter and milder in flavor than regular brown whole wheat flour, resembling all-purpose flour after baking. Use the same as whole wheat pastry flour.

OTHER WHOLE-GRAIN FLOURS: Lots of whole-grain flours are becoming more common on grocery store shelves, and they can be great when you want to whip up a more nutritious batch of cookies. Oat flour is what it sounds like, flour made from oats. We like to use a touch of oat flour with wheat flour to create a pleasantly grainy texture. Brown rice flour has no gluten at all so unless you're going for

---

★ ★ ★

THE ALL-PURPOSE FLOUR MYSTERY

Not all all-purpose flours are created equal—this can become apparent even when baking cookies. From coast to coast, north to south, or country to country, flours will vary ever so slightly in moisture and protein content. Sometimes your cookies will be higher or flatter or softer than other times (even when you're sure you did everything right). Typically this has a lot to do with the composition of the flour, how you measure it, and even the weather. See our Troubleshooting tips on page 30. As a general guideline, we recommend using standard, unbleached, all-purpose flours for well-structured cookies. Do not use "cake"-type white flours as they are low protein and may unexpectedly sabotage all your hard cookie work.

gluten-free baking (see our gluten-free tips below), you'll need to blend it with wheat flours to get properly formed cookies. Other favorite nonwheat flours of ours include quinoa and millet. Both have their own particular taste and texture ... try substituting ½ to ¾ cup for all-purpose flour in recipes and see if you like their unique flavors.

* * *

HOW TO MAKE YOUR COOKIES GLUTEN-FREE
(GLUTEN-FREE IS NOT A COOKIE DEATH SENTENCE)

Cheer up, Mr. Gloomypants, and step away from the ledge. Just because you can't have gluten doesn't mean you have to be left out of the milk and cookies party. In fact, this might be the beginning of an all-out adventure. There is such a variety of flour available these days that sometimes the hardest part of living gluten-free is deciding which ones to use. The tastes and textures of these flours are so interesting and yummy that sometimes we go gluten-free just for fun. But, ya know, we also organize our spice rack for fun, so take that with a grain of salt.

So here's a news flash: any of the cookies in this book can be made gluten-free. Yeah, we said it. There are a few gluten-free-specific recipes in these pages, but the reason there isn't a big whopping GF chapter is because cookies are so flexible, subbing in gluten-free flour is a breeze.

The basic trick is that gluten-free flours across the board absorb liquid differently than all-purpose flour, so a bit of tweaking of the amount of flour is necessary. Generally, we use up to ¼ cup more gluten-free flour per cup of all-purpose flour. If you're using a store-bought gluten-free mix, it may say that it's a 1:1 swap, but we suggest adding at least 2 tablespoons more to improve the structure of your cookies. Our gluten-free mix already makes that swap, so use as directed.

Isa & Terry's Gluten Frida Mix

Even though the flours in this recipe add up to more than a cup, use this ratio 1:1 per cup of flour. If you can't find these flours at your health food store, they are all available from Bob's Red Mill (www.bobsredmill.com). When choosing between coconut and almond flour, know that these flours do taste like the nuts they come from, so decide which you're in the mood for. When choosing between quinoa and millet flour, know that quinoa costs three times as much—that might help you decide! Store gluten-free flours in the fridge to keep them as fresh as possible.

¼ cup almond flour or coconut flour
⅓ cup white rice flour
⅓ cup quinoa flour or millet flour
3 tablespoons tapioca flour
1 tablespoon ground flax seeds

* * *

WHOLE GRAINS

OATMEAL is probably the most famous whole grain (as in actual whole seed with bran and germ intact), making a much-beloved appearance in oatmeal cookies. We like to experiment with the subtle difference between delicate quick-cooking oats and hearty, chewy old-fashioned rolled oats. Beyond oats, most other uncooked grains are too tough to just toss into cookie dough.

SWEETENERS

Probably the second most important ingredient in any cookie is a sweetener. Lucky for us, in this modern age we have a vast array of sweeteners ranging from the pristine, minimally refined to the classic, easy-to-use white variety. Choosing the right sweetener can strongly influence the flavor and texture of your cookie, so check out our substitute section before sacrificing that cup of maple syrup to the cookie gods. When we call for sugar in a recipe, we mean either granulated white sugar or evaporated cane juice, unless otherwise noted.

GRANULATED WHITE SUGAR: Everyone knows granulated white sugar as plain old sugar. There's plenty of discussion (any Internet search will do) about the vegan-ness of white table sugar because sometimes it is processed with the aid of animal bone char. To eliminate any doubts, look for organic sugar. We like to use granulated white sugar in baked goods because there are great vegan options available these days. It's also still the cheapest sweetener and easy to use with predictable results. Whole Foods now carries its own packaged vegan sugar, handily labeled as such and in bountiful 4-pound bags.

Another popular brand of organic vegan sugar is Florida Crystals.

It's also worth noting that if sugar is made from sugar beets instead of cane sugar, it will always be processed in a vegan way, but it can be tricky determining whether sugar is from beet or cane. But you know, don't let any of this confuse you. You probably know what sugar is so just go ahead and go read something more important now, like that 800-page biography on Robert Moses.

DEMERARA SUGAR: We love to use this large grain sugar for decorating. It's a less refined cane sugar, so some of the cane's natural golden hue is preserved. Because the crystals are larger, they will hold their shape, giving baked cookies a sparkly, disco-like appearance.

EVAPORATED CANE JUICE: You can use evaporated cane juice wherever we call for sugar. It acts exactly the same in recipes, but it is processed a bit less and retains some of its vitamins. Because when you're eating cookies what you're really thinking about is vitamins. Evaporated cane juice is usually available in health food stores.

BROWN SUGAR: The darling of cinnamony treats, brown sugar is just white sugar that has been flavored and moistened with a touch of molasses. It adds delectable, buttery flavor to vegan cookies. We use dark brown sugar in these recipes, but you may use light if that's what floats your boat.

SUCANAT is a dry, natural sweetener, popular with the healthy baking crowd, and when we first started vegan baking it was the only game in town. Its funny-sounding name isn't from an alien language, it's actually an abbreviation for "sugar cane natural." We call specifically for Sucanat in a few recipes, such as the 21ST-CENTURY CAROB CHIP COOKIES (page 94), where we want a hint of molasses flavor in a less processed format than brown sugar. Essentially, it's the juice from sugar cane that has been dried but, unlike regular white sugar, it has not had its nutrients zapped to kingdom come. You can use Sucanat to replace the sugar in a recipe but note that it will result in a molasses taste, which is great if that's what you're going for. It also makes the product a bit more cakey than sugar does. You don't necessarily have to time travel back to the 1970s for Sucanat; it's generally available in modern-day health food stores.

MOLASSES is a slightly less processed liquid sugar cane product that adds a special dark color and flavor to baked goods. Regular molasses is generally used in these recipes when molasses is called for. Blackstrap molasses (used, for example, in BLACKSTRAP GINGER-SNAPS, page 42) is thicker, darker, and less sweet with a complex, bittersweet flavor.

PURE MAPLE SYRUP has become insanely expensive so we don't really rely on it much, but it does work great in mixing up a vegan chocolate ganache! And sometimes you just need that special maple flavor. Look for darker, slightly less pricy Grade B syrup to use in baked goods. Grade B actually has a stronger maple flavor than Grade A, so it's a case of more for just a bit less. Never use that Aunt Jemima or Mrs. Butterworth stuff—it's just artificially flavored high-fructose corn syrup.

BROWN RICE SYRUP: The name doesn't sound like much but don't let it fool you; brown rice syrup is a delectable natural liquid sweetener made from whole-grain rice. Thick and rich and caramel-like, you'd never guess it's still a whole food. Not overly sweet, too, so we use it in a few wholesome cookies and for recipes that need extra ooey-gooey tastiness.

AGAVE NECTAR: The latest sweet darling in the health food scene, agave is made from the cooked sap of the succulent agave plant. It's intensely sweet, even more so than white sugar. It's reported to have a minimal impact on blood sugar levels, making it diabetic-friendly, but we like it for its clean, light taste.

BARLEY MALT is a thick, mildly sweet, molasses-like liquid that packs a punch of rich, toasted malted barley flavor. We like to use it in combination with other natural sweeteners (agave or maple) to temper its intense flavor. We call for it in only one or two recipes, so don't throw your grocer up against a wall demanding to know where it is until you're sure you're going to need it.

FATS

Oils, margarine, and shortening bring the flavor and tenderness to baked goods, and cookies are no exception. Cookies in general tend to have a higher ratio of fat (and sugar) to flour than less "dessert-y" baked goods (scones, muffins), just to give you an idea of

***

NONDAIRY MILK

Because cookies don't generally require a whole lot of milk, the kind you use is pretty much up to you. None of these cookies call for a specific kind of milk, although you should stick to plain or unsweetened varieties or vanilla if you must. Some of our favorite vegan milks include soy, rice, and almond.

how important fats are to achieving yummy cookies. The less fat a cookie has the moister and cakier it tastes; if you've ever replaced oil with applesauce in a recipe you'll know what we mean.

CANOLA AND OTHER VEGETABLE OILS: A healthy, easy-to-find, and cost-effective choice, canola is our general "go-to" in baking, with its neutral taste, healthy nutritional profile, and even a little bit of Omega 3s. Look for minimally processed, preferably cold-pressed. If canola oil isn't your thing, feel free to try other light-tasting oils such as sunflower, safflower, or even plain old "vegetable oil."

MARGARINE: Not just any old margarine, margarine without trans fats or hydrogenation should be your goal when ingredient shopping. As of this writing, Earth Balance seems to be the most popular vegan margarine in the United States that is also both nonhydrogenated and trans fat–free. This ain't your grandma's margarine. In fact, the company doesn't even call it margarine, that is much too gauche! It's simply a "buttery spread." Read labels and check that there are no dairy products (whey, dairy solids, etc.) hidden within, or look for a visit from the vegan police.

SHORTENING: A great American baking ingredient that creates cookies with a firm texture and provides a reliable baking experience. Just like with margarine, it pays to be picky. There are now several excellent organic shortenings available that are both nonhydrogenated and free of pesky trans fats. Earth Balance shortening and margarine is also available in a convenient baking stick form.

COCONUT OIL: Natural unhydrogenated coconut oil has become increasingly popular and is an interesting option in cooking and baking. We don't call for it too much because it can get pretty pricy. Use only unhydrogenated coconut oil in these recipes, either refined (neutral-scented) or unrefined (richly coconut-scented). Coconut oil has the notable property of remaining semisolid at room temperature and becoming very firm if chilled. We like to use it semisolid (easy to scoop) or melted. There is some controversy about the healthfulness of this oil; some claim it cures whatever ails you, others claim it is the food of the devil. We will just step aside from all that and munch on our biscotti since the information will probably change by the time this book is in print.

NUT BUTTERS AND FRUIT PRESERVES

Nut butters turn ordinary cookie dough into delectable treats. Fruit preserves can be baked on top of cookies for a pretty gem-like effect or used to glue two unsuspecting cookies together for a tasty little sandwich. Have a good selection of both and you'll never be at a loss for making everyday cookies something special.

We always use **NATURAL PEANUT BUTTER** in our recipes to avoid the nasty stuff full of hydrogenated oils. Be sure to stir any separated oil back into natural peanut butter before measuring for recipes. Since natural peanut butters can vary in moisture and oil content from brand to brand (and even batch to batch) you may have to make certain adjustments with the recipes. If your cookie dough seems too dry, add a tablespoon or two of nondairy milk. In the unlikely event the dough looks way too soupy, sprinkle in a tablespoon of flour.

PEANUT, ALMOND, AND HAZELNUT BUTTERS prove that you can find most any kind

★ ★ ★

WHAT IS PH BALANCE & WHAT THE PH DOES IT HAVE TO DO WITH COOKIES?

We bet that as you nodded out in chemistry class and drooled all over your textbook you never imagined your little nap would affect your cookie baking. Ph is simply how acidic (or not) a substance is. The less acidic a substance is, the more alkaline, or "basic," it is.

of nut converted into a spreadable form these days. Peanut butter baked goods are always a crowd-pleaser, and we're no exception to the masses; see PEANUT BUTTER BLONDIES (page 129) and PEANUT BUTTER CRISSCROSSES (page 81), just to name a few examples. If you can't do peanuts, toasted soy nut butter is a great alternative. Almond and hazelnut butters are luxurious and nutritious other-butters; try some in HAZELNUT FUDGE DREAMIES (page 176).

FRUIT JAMS AND JELLIES: It's really up to you what to use on top of delicate thumbprint cookies or slathered between any drop or rolled cookie. For best results, we recommend using the thickest preserves you can get, such as a good chunky strawberry jam or a dense orange marmalade. Also great for cookies are raspberry (with or without seeds), blackberry, and blueberry preserves. For a different kind of preserve cookie, try CRAN-BERRY WALNUT THUMBPRINTS (page 153) if you've run out of things to do with post-Thanksgiving jellied cranberry sauce. Always be sure to give your jams a good stir before using to incorporate any water that might have pooled to the top and to achieve maximum spreadability.

STARCHES

Starches are that little something extra we like to include for texture. Sometimes starches step in for the special binding properties of eggs in vegan goodies or are added to create a special crisp lightness.

Cornstarch, a highly refined starch, can create cookies that are both delicate and slightly chewy. Arrowroot powder may be the most expensive of the three but blends seamlessly into cookie dough. This ground powder of a tropical root has properties similar to cornstarch, and we use them interchangeably. Tapioca flour, also sometimes packaged as tapioca starch, will give baked goods a chewier texture. We will let you know which of these starches works best in any given recipe.

COCOA POWDER AND SEMISWEET CHOCOLATE

Of course we have to talk about chocolate, because we're certain you came here looking for chocolaty cookies. Cocoa powder is the easiest way to make satisfying chocolate baked treats. We only use unsweetened cocoa powder in these recipes, so save the sugar-added stuff for making hot chocolate.

DUTCH-PROCESSED COCOA: "Dutched" chocolate has undergone a Ph-altering process, resulting in mellow-but-complex chocolate flavor and deepening of the chocolate's color. We call specifically for Dutch-processed cocoa in many recipes, and popular brands like Droste are available in well-stocked supermarkets.

UNSWEETENED COCOA POWDER: This is what you'll see most often in the baking section—your standard Hershey's or Ghirardelli is just good old unsweetened cocoa powder. It has a light color and a pure chocolate taste.

BLACK COCOA POWDER: This is a specialty cocoa that adds an even deeper color and bittersweet chocolate notes to baked goods. Black cocoa powder is made when cocoa is "super" Dutch-processed until it reaches a black, sooty color (though it doesn't have the most intense chocolate flavor). Never use only black cocoa powder in a recipe; just a few tablespoons combined with regular cocoa powder create an ideal blend of rich dark "Oreo" color and chocolate flavor.

SEMISWEET CHOCOLATE: For extra-smooth chocolate depth, we occasionally use melted semisweet chocolate. See ESPRESSO FUDGE BROWNIES (page 130) for the uses and wonderful effects of a little melted chocolate in a vegan brownie! In chip or square form, semisweet chocolate makes cookies extra rich and moist by delivering cocoa butter's excellent texture to your baked goods.

With most any chocolate products, you get what you pay for. Sure, that Prada knockoff clutch purse looks fine, but you don't have to eat it. Cheap chocolate and cocoa powder taste cheap, and nobody wants to be educated about your inner cheapskate by biting into your homemade brownies. More expensive, higher-quality brands will make an impact. Since vegan goods go without the ingredients that usually flavor recipes (namely butter and eggs), this is something to consider, so feel good about spending a little extra on chocolate (and extracts, too) when you're baking to impress!

CHOCOLATE CHIPS AND FRIENDS

Chocolate chips are about as iconic a cookie ingredient as one can get. Perhaps the biggest thing to look for when shopping for chips is to insure you're buying a vegan product sans dairy ingredients such as butter oil, whey, or nonfat dried milk solids. Luckily there are more and more excellent vegan chips out there. What we said about buying quality chocolate generally rings true here, too, but sometimes you can get away with slightly less spendy chips if the rest of your ingredients are top notch (but don't get carried away, Cheapy McCheapster!).

Chocolate chips come in all kinds of varieties these days, our go-to chip being semisweet. Bittersweet works, too, it just has a lower sugar content than semisweet and it's a bit harder to find vegan bittersweet chips. Chocolate chunks are a fun alterna-chip when you want to bite into a big mouthful of chocolate. On the other hand, sometimes adorable mini chocolate chips are just the thing to elevate your tiny little cookies to the supercute stratosphere. For the longest time, vegan white chocolate chips were impossible to come by, but now you can just pay a visit to a good online vegan boutique or even a kosher grocery (see notes on shopping, beginning on page 19). Another hard-to-come-by-but-worth-the-search chip is accidentally vegan butterscotch chips that come alive (in

a yummy, not creepy zombie way) in oatmeal cookies. Look for them in large supermarket chains, often re-labeled as the "generic" supermarket brand. Sometimes other exciting twists on vegan chips such as vegan chocolate coffee chips show up online, so grab 'em while they're hot.

No discussion of cookie candy chips is complete without carob chips. The famous old-school un-chocolate is really something to be experienced so why not give it a try in 21ST-CENTURY CAROB CHIP COOKIES (page 94). Just be sure to read the ingredients to check for vegan-ness; sometimes carob chips contain nonfat dry milk or other dairy solids.

NUTS AND SEEDS

Nuts and seeds of all kinds are all favorite mix-ins to cookies. Grated coconut, either sweetened flake or unsweetened dried, gives a lot of texture to cookies (similar in bulk to oatmeal) along with that unmistakable coconut flavor. The easiest way to add nuts to any cookie is to roughly chop them (using a chef's knife is ideal for controlling the size of nut pieces) and fold them in toward the end. Chopped walnuts, peanuts, macadamias,

"BUT WHAT DO YOU USE INSTEAD OF *EGGS?*"

THIS MAY BE the second-most common question after, "But where do you get your protein?" when the topic of eating vegan comes up. Here's an idea ... make those questioners a batch of cookies and they'll marvel at how baking is possible beyond the chicken and the egg. There are several things we use to replace eggs in baking, and we switch it up depending on the desired flavor or texture.

We love to use ground flax seeds to help hold together dense cookie dough loaded with whole grains, nuts, or chips. Cornstarch or arrowroot/tapioca flour binds more delicate cookies. Sometimes we just leave it out and let the gluten in the flour or the melding of baked sugar and fats do all the work. What we don't require are the premixed powdered vegan "egg substitutes" sometimes used in vegan baking. They're just a blend of starches anyway and require mixing with water. Why buy yet another ingredient when you can just as easily get the same effects with the stuff you probably already have in your pantry?

pecans, almonds, and hazelnuts are at home in most any cookie. Occasionally we grind up almonds, pecans, or walnuts with a food processor and mix them into dough to create a fine crumb and rich, nutty flavor. We store nuts in the fridge to keep them fresh, and sometimes even in the freezer if we've got a metric ton that we won't be finishing off anytime soon.

A few seeds show up in these recipes. Ground flax seeds appear frequently but for reasons other than might be expected. When ground flax is beaten with a little liquid, it forms a viscous gel that conveniently behaves much like eggs and can provide binding and structure in cookies. Especially useful when cookie dough contains plenty of chunky ingredients (oats, fruits) or whole-grain flour.

For the best-looking results we like to use ground golden flax seed (also called flax seed meal) because the color blends in seamlessly, like a ninja in the night.

Sesame seeds, poppy seeds, pumpkin seeds (pepitas), or sunflower seeds are great additions for boosting flavor, crunch, and nutrition, too!

DRIED FRUIT

Here's another mix-in item you can experiment with in any given cookie recipe without much effect on baking chemistry. So what we're saying here is that if you're a raisin-hater (why, we don't know), try substituting dried cranberries. Some of our favorites that typically go into cookies: raisins of all kinds (Thompson, golden, red flame) and dried cranberries, cherries, apricots, papaya, figs, apples, and pineapple, chopped as needed to get morsel-size bits.

EXTRACTS

It's been said many times many ways: buy the best-quality extracts you can afford. Since vegan baked goods forgo animal products, ex-

tracts play a vital role in flavoring up your goodies. You can't go wrong by investing in a big bottle of pure vanilla extract, so read that label carefully and avoid artificial vanilla (also known as vanillin). And almond extract is not just for almond-flavored things anymore! It adds sweetly nutty, fruity notes to chocolate baked goods and more depth to plain old vanilla ones. Beyond that there's a whole paradise of extracts to choose from ... most of the time we use them in addition to vanilla to round out the entire flavor profile of any given cookie. Some of our favorite extracts include: chocolate, coffee, lemon, orange, mint, maple, and coconut.

LEAVENING AGENTS

Important for creating volume, baking powder and baking soda are essential to most recipes. The most crucial thing is to make sure you're not using a batch of either that's so old you don't remember when you bought it, as leavening agents slowly lose their chemical strength over time. Cream of tartar is an old-fashioned leavening agent that isn't used much anymore, but we like to use it in CITY GIRL SNICKERDOODLES (page 46) for nostalgia's sake.

SALT

Even sweets need a dash of salt to enliven and balance out flavors. Regular old table salt is just fine for baking, as is fine-ground sea salt. Once in a while a dash of fancy gourmet salt—like fleur de sel—makes a difference if sprinkled very lightly on top of cookies, as in CARAMEL PECAN BARS (page 111), for the exciting variation of SALTED CARAMEL PECAN BARS (page 113)!

LET'S GO SHOPPING ONLINE!

Shopping online for ingredients—either hard-to-find vegan items or specialty baking stuff—makes more sense than ever. Below are a few of our favorite resources. Whether you live in the country or the middle of a bustling metropolis, you'll love the convenience and selection.

Baker's Catalogue at King Arthur Flour

bakerscatalogue.com
Get your black cocoa powder and delightful Dutch and natural cocoa powder blends here along with specialty high-quality flavor extracts, espresso powder, and top-notch baking tools. They also sell the coveted mini-chocolate chip.

Bob's Red Mill

bobsredmill.com
It's no secret we love Bob's vast selection of whole-grain flours and freshly ground flax seeds. Everything from whole wheat pastry to gluten-free blends are at your disposal.

Food Fight! Vegan Grocery

foodfightgrocery.com
Home to vegan white chocolate chips and puffy vegan marshmallows!

Pangea Vegan Store

veganstore.com
Pangea carries their own brand of vegan white chocolate chips along with other vegan baking supplies.

SHOPPING WITH PANTS: OFF-LINE SHOPPING

Vegan baking is one of those things that usually requires a special in-person shopping trip now and then.

We recommend first getting familiar with

your local vegan-friendly food co-op or health food store if you haven't already to make shopping for supplies all the easier. If you're just starting your vegan-baking shopping voyage and aren't sure where to go in your neighborhood, websites like greenpeople.org or a few Google searches are helpful. Okay, it's not totally off-line shopping anymore, but what do you expect in this day 'n' age?

Whole Foods Market carries their own brand of specially labeled vegan and fair-trade sugar and vegan chocolate chips. They're also a mostly reliable source of vegan, nonhydrogenated Earth Balance shortening and buttery baking sticks. As long as you can resist spending your entire paycheck here you're doing just fine.

The hunt for vegan butterscotch chips, a favorite topic on the vegan Internet (see it to believe it), can actually yield results if you happen to live near a Food Lion or Price Chopper supermarket (in the eastern part of the United States). As of this writing these national chains carry accidentally vegan butterscotch baking chips, typically branded as the generic store brand. Since they're chock full of not-too-great hydrogenated oils, we don't recommend eating these every day (or every other), but a handful tossed into any oatmeal cookie in this book (hint hint, COWBOY COOKIES, page 48) can be a fun special-occasion treat. Be sure to always read ingredients, though, as these things can change in our crazy, mixed-up world.

Kosher grocery stores (both online and off) can also be interesting places to find more accidentally vegan candies and chocolate chips. Look for products labeled Parve (or Pareve/Parevine) for starters to insure dairy-free. Since online stores may not list ingredients on their websites, an in-person shopping trip (plus some ingredient label reading) can help you locate vegan chocolate chips, sometimes even in fun flavors such as coffee and mint.

TOOLS FOR SUCCESS
(For Achieving Cookies, That Is)

OF ALL THE THINGS you will bake in your life, cookies probably require the least amount of equipment and preparation. It's why kids, moms, college students, and busy people worldwide turn to making cookies when the need for something sweet arises. Here's what kitchen supplies you'll need—you may even have all of this stuff already. If that's the case, check out our Something Extras list (page 22) for other things that make cookie baking even easier and less fussy, if that's possible.

THE ESSENTIALS

These are the bare necessities for making the simplest cookie of all, the drop cookie. If "minimalist baker" is what you write on your tax forms, then all you really need are the following things to mix dough in and bake cookies on.

COOKIE SHEETS come in all shapes, materials, and sizes these days. Our favorite cookie sheets are the thin aluminum kind with one slightly raised edge for grasping on to, but use whatever style appeals to you and your budget. Consider using those thick **double-insulated sheets** if your oven is prone to hot spots or your cookies turn too brown on the bottom too fast no matter what you do (see the info on oven thermometers, page 25, though!). We like to use the light metal sheets, since darker metal is more prone to burning your precious little cookie bottoms.

MIXING BOWLS and **MIXING UTENSILS** are what you make them, but we recommend you invest in quality stainless steel or plastic bowls in various sizes. You'll be happier than if you mixed your cookie dough in a cereal bowl. A **wire whisk** is perfect for emulsifying liquid ingredients (such as nondairy milk with oil), and **wooden spoons** and **rubber spatulas** are great for mixing in dry ingredients and folding in things like rolled oats or chocolate chips. A **large fork** or specialized pastry fork makes fast work of creaming solid fats by hand when you need only a little for a frosting or filling. And, truthfully, most of these cookies can be mixed using nothing but a god-given fork.

ALUMINUM FOIL should be on every list for anything ever. You always need it for something. In this case, lining pans when the recipe calls for it.

THIN METAL or **PLASTIC BAKING SPATU-LAS** not only make lifting finished cookies off baking sheets a breeze but also work wonders when moving delicate rolled cookie dough onto baking sheets.

OVEN MITTS are not to be forgotten when moving hot cookie sheets out of and back into a hot oven! In a pinch use a folded **thick kitchen towel.**

PARCHMENT PAPER may at first not seem like an essential tool, but once you get used to the ease, mess reduction, and never-sticking results, it's difficult to go back to greasing (and cleaning) baking sheets. One piece of paper can typically survive being baked several times or the amount needed for an average cookie recipe. Never ever substitute waxed paper for parchment paper!

THE SOMETHING EXTRAS

When your needs go beyond basic drop cookies, these apparent "extra" supplies will go the long haul for dozens and dozens of great rolled or sliced cookies and bars. Soon some of these could become essential to you.

BROWNIE AND BAR COOKIE PANS are what you need if brownies or bar cookies are what you want. The classic 8 x 8-inch brownie pan is indispensable and is ideally suited for all the brownies and blondies in this book— using a larger pan can produce cookies with less than optimal results. For other bar-type cookies, we like to use a 9 x 13-inch pan. Bars made with this kind of pan can be sliced into either sixteen generously sized portions or twenty-four petite cookies. For the record, we always recommend using metal pans for vegan baking, as glass or silicon pans can create soggy baked goods that rise unevenly.

COOKIE DOUGH SCOOPERS, also called "dishers," make dishing cookie dough onto baking sheets almost too easy. A little like old-fashioned ice cream scoops, cookie dough scoops can be purchased in varying sizes from jumbo to teeny teaspoon size and insure consistently shaped and sized drop cookies. And of course you can use these for ice cream: they're the perfect multifunction tool! Use either nonstick spray or a light sprinkle of water to keep dough from sticking to scoops.

COOLING RACKS are another cookie baking item that's hard to avoid once you get used to using them. Cooling cookies on these metal wire racks (instead of just leaving them to cool on cookie sheets) insures crisp cookie bottoms without a hint of sogginess. Plus they're a convenient parking place for freshly baked goods. Well-made cooling racks have extendable fold-out "legs" so that racks can be stacked to save valuable counter space.

A HANDHELD MIXER is what you'll need for making lots of fluffy frostings and creamy cookie fillings quickly and easily. It doesn't even have to be an expensive one; a $12 hand mixer will quickly pay for itself after whipping up few batches of frosting or creaming mounds of margarine and shortening. **Rubber spatulas** are handy tools, too, when working dough with your hand mixer.

FLOUR SIFTERS do the job when it comes to sifting flour, cocoa powder, and other powdery additions like baking soda and baking powder. The most common style available is shaped a like a big beer mug with metal mesh on the bottom and moving parts in the handle that do the sifting work. If you prefer, use a **fine-gauge wire mesh strainer** instead, balancing the rim and handle on the edge of your mixing bowl. Just give the sides of the sifter a gentle tap to sift the flour into the bowl!

FROSTING SPATULAS look a little like spackling knives and make frosting the tops of cookies fast and easy.

PASTRY BAGS AND DECORATING TIPS help make those pretty frosted holiday cookies happen. If you're just beginning, look for low-cost kits that include a bag and a few plastic tips. Advanced cookie decorators like to have a wide assortment of high-quality metal tips and reusable canvas pastry bags. We also like very large tips for pressing out soft cookie dough when making specialty cookies like STARRY FUDGE SHORTBREAD (page 167).

DOUBLE BOILERS and MICROWAVE-SAFE BOWLS are your two options when it comes to melting chocolate for dipping, decorating, and brownie making. Double boilers are old-school stovetop setups. They consist of a set of fitted glass pots that safely melt chocolate without the risk of burning it. You can also fake this setup by resting a small pan inside a larger one filled with enough water to cover the bottom of smaller pan, but not so much that it will overflow. An easier, faster way to melt chocolate is in a microwave. Heat chocolate in a microwave-safe glass bowl for 1 to 1½ minutes at 60 percent heat (low power)—just enough to make chips soft and easily form a melted mass when stirred. Because it can burn so easily, never use high microwave power when melting chocolate.

COOKIE CUTTERS are a no-brainer if you're a dedicated cookie-decorating enthusiast. Metal cutters can last forever but plastic cutters are a cheap and plentiful option. A quick Internet search will reveal a bewildering range of cookie cutter shapes from adorable (squirrels, penguins, hummingbirds) to sassy (mermaids, flamingos, chili peppers) to cryptic (a tooth, toothbrush, pliers … a cautionary reminder?). There are even "make your own" kits available out there if you look hard enough. In general, we tend to avoid cutters that feature too many thin spindly bits as these parts may brown faster than the main body of the cookie. Simple, scalloped-edge round cutters are good all-purpose cookie cutters that can be used all year round, not just on holidays or National Rocketship-Shaped Cookie day.

COOKIE SPRITZ KITS are unavoidable if you love spritz cookies, the rich little shortbread cookie pressed into cute flower- or star-shaped patterns. The STARRY FUDGE SHORTBREAD (page 167) dough works great in whatever cookie spritz device you like. Better kits will come with plenty of easily switched plates in decorative shapes that you can use for any occasion.

OVEN THERMOMETERS TO THE RESCUE

YOUR OVEN IS YOUR FRIEND. Usually. All too often, older home ovens can be temperamental and prone to uneven heating, or even worse, never being at the temperature your stove dial claims. If your oven is a dishonest sort you may already suspect it: burned cookie bottoms or baked goods that seem either very underdone or way overcooked when the estimated baking time has been reached. If that's the case, you are in desperate need of an oven thermometer! They are inexpensive, and if you learn to use one, it's as good as getting a new oven, almost.

Use only oven thermometers designed to be placed *inside* the oven and built to withstand those high temperatures. Follow the manufacturer's directions or just place the thermometer in the center oven rack before preheating the oven, leaving the thermometer to gauge what's going on as the heat rises. The average oven requires about 20 to 22 minutes to preheat so take a peek around then to get an idea if your oven is being truthful. If things are wildly off, you may need to let the oven heat longer or bring the dial down a notch. Recheck the temperature every 8 to 10 minutes until your desired temperature is reached.

★ ★ ★

THE SCIENCE OF COOKIES
CRITERIA FOR CONSUMMATE COOKIES

Cookie baking is pretty straightforward, so chances are you will follow the recipes and your cookies will come out magnificently. However, there are a few golden rules to insure fabulousness every time.

❖ **Make sure your oven is at the right temperature.** We don't want to sound like a broken record, but your heat source is the king in baking. If you're not positive how accurate your oven is, get an oven thermometer (see page 25). Always preheat your oven as directed and remember to set a timer so that you don't just plumb forget how long the cookies have been in.

❖ **Use the proper pans.** Clean, aluminum baking sheets either lined with parchment or lightly greased (as the recipe directs) is the way to go. Don't rely on a glass pan, or a hubcap, or a piece of aluminum foil, for that matter.

❖ **Don't overcrowd the oven.** We often just bake one sheet of cookies at a time. Even putting two sheets of cookies in at the same time can result in uneven baking. You know the boundaries of your oven best, and if you don't, then get to know them. See what your oven can and can't handle and play it safe.

❖ **You got to know when to hold 'em and know when to fold 'em.** Knowing if a cookie is underbaked or overbaked takes a little experience. With drop cookies especially, they might appear to be underbaked when you follow the recipe cooking times, but remember that cookies are still baking a little as they cool on the baking sheet. The texture also changes drastically as it cools. Check that the bottoms are slightly browned; that is a good test for doneness. And the tops of cookies should not be firm (unless the recipe says so)—that means they're overbaked.

❖ **Make cookies consistently sized.** Check out our tools section for information about cookie dishers (page 23); you don't have to break out the food scale and be perfect about it, but aim for the same amount of dough in each cookie so that they bake at the same rate.

★ ★ ★

SUBSTITUTING
Some Tough Love for Trying Cookie Times

THE BEST DAY of school was always when your Spanish teacher was out sick and in came the sub. You would throw school equipment out the window, lock other students in the janitor's closet, and deal Quaaludes right from your desk, right? Then one day a different kind of substitute arrived. Just as you were going to clean erasers on a classmate's head, she used some sort of wizardry to hurl you back into your seat. Before you knew it, you were writing a 5,000-word essay extolling the virtues of the Chilean coastline.

The point is, not all substitutes are created equal. Every so often (when we're Googling ourselves twenty-five times a day) we'll find someone complaining that their cookies came out wrong. All they did was replace the oil with jelly and the chocolate chips with bubblegum, or something like that. Now, we're no strangers to invention. We've opened the pantry and gotten the bad news, too: *out of brown sugar*. Sometimes subbing is necessary and any home baker would do well to know how to make those changes successfully. Whether it's because you want gluten-free goodies for your nephew or you just came into a sandbag of almond flour, we've got you covered.

Flours are probably the most common substitutes made. It's okay to do, but just know what you're getting into.

ALL-PURPOSE FLOUR

Swap with: **whole wheat pastry flour, white whole wheat flour,** or ISA & TERRY'S GLUTEN FRIDA MIX (see page 8) The taste and texture will be more grainy and slightly more dry. Try swapping out only half the flour called for to up the nutrition without messing with the taste and texture too much.

MARGARINE

Swap with: **vegetable oil.** It's a sad day when you go for that tub o' Earth Balance and the container is light as a feather with nothing but a spoonful of the buttery stuff. That simply won't do. You can sub vegetable oil, like canola, for the margarine in many recipes. We don't suggest it for shortbread-type recipes, where you're really depending on a buttery flavor and melt-in-your-mouth texture, but for drop cookies, sure, why not? The texture will be a bit more cakey and the cookie will spread a bit less. Always use a little less oil than margarine. If the recipe calls for ½ cup of margarine, use around ⅓ cup of oil.

FAT IN GENERAL

Swap with: **applesauce.** If you're looking to make your cookie lower in fat in general, ap-plesauce is your friend. For ½ cup of oil or margarine, use ⅓ cup of applesauce plus a tablespoon of oil. The cookie will be much softer and, uh, not as good. But at least it will be super-low in fat!

SUGAR

Swap with: **Sucanat or liquid sweeteners** (like agave or maple syrup) if you must. Often, people want to replace plain old sugar in a recipe with something a little healthier. We hear you. Now if only we could watch you! This sub can be difficult to make. You can do a 1:1 sub with Sucanat without too much trouble.

But what if you want to use agave to make your cookies diabetic-friendly, or maple syrup because you love Vermont? The dry-to-liquid substitution is super-tricky and not all that consistent. We make it sometimes, but we're seasoned professionals living that close to danger at all times. Instead, we suggest you use an already agave-sweetened recipe (like the ORANGE AGAVE CHOCOLATE CHIP COOKIES recipe, page 98) and modify the flavors of that recipe as needed. However, you might still want to sub stuff as much as we warn against it, so at least we can provide you with the info you need to help you on your way.

Basically what you want to do is lower the rest of the liquid ingredients and increase the dry without upsetting the balance too much. If the recipe calls for 1 cup of sugar, use only ¾ of maple or agave. Leave any milk out of the recipe. Now just add tablespoons of flour until it seems to be a good cookie consistency. We know. Not at all a science. Try not to do it.

BROWN SUGAR

Swap with: **sugar plus molasses.** For each ½ cup of brown sugar, remove 2 tablespoons sugar and add 2 teaspoons molasses. No big whoop.

PEANUT BUTTER

Swap with: **other nut butters.** If you have a peanut allergy and a penchant for almonds, then use these nut butters interchangeably. You can also sub any other nut butter, if you're a millionaire. Cashew butter and macadamia butter and the like tend to be super-expensive. Soy nut butter is cheap enough, so that could be worth investigating.

FLAX SEEDS

Swap with: **starch.** Usually flax seeds are there for texture and structure, so look at it the same way you would look at replacing eggs. Add a bit of starch, about half the amount of flax seed called for.

STARCH

Swap with: **tapioca, cornstarch, arrowroot.** Different starches act in different ways. Tapioca tends to make goods a bit chewier, and cornstarch and arrowroot provide more crispness. But they all do the job of holding the whole party together, so we use them interchangeably.

TROUBLESHOOTING

Something Wicked Comes to the Cookie Sheet

BAKING COOKIES should be as simple as eating raw cookie dough. Usually it is, but sometimes a little extra know-how can be the difference between bottom-burnt hockey pucks and the kind of treats that get asked for again and again. It's important to note that the mood swings of flour are often the culprit here. Through no fault of our own, flour can be affected by humidity and elevation, in addition to which it simply varies from brand to brand. Here are some of the most common cookie disasters—and how to prevent them.

EXHIBIT A: *Dough is crumbly and dry*

Suspect: Too much flour. Did you accidentally sneak an extra cup of flour into the recipe while we weren't looking? Of course not, but we're going to have to use our flour extraction lasers to remove some of that flour. Or ...

Solution: You can add a few tablespoons of nondairy milk until the mixture resembles cookie dough and not a sandy beach. Careful about mixing the liquid in, especially if the dough's got starch in it, as you don't want the cookies to become gummy. Use your hands to mix it in. Be firm but gentle!

EXHIBIT B: *They spread too much*

Suspect: Too much liquid. Instead of nice individual cookies, do you have one uniform mass of Frankencookie? The dough is too wet. Even though we have meticulously tested all of the recipes, flour can be a temperamental mistress. Experience will let you know when a cookie dough is just too darn wet, but unless the recipe says otherwise, cookie dough should not spread out like a pancake on your sheet.

Solution: Add a few extra tablespoons of flour to correct the situation.

EXHIBIT C: *They don't spread enough*

Suspect: Too much flour

Solution: Again, this is a job for extra unmilk. Get to adding.

EXHIBIT D: *Burnt bottoms*

Suspect #1: Your oven. It could be hot spots (not the kind you'd want to be seen at). Are your cookies turning up pale on one of the sheet but overly browned on the other? You then have a case of the "uneven oven": heat that is not evenly distributed can lead to spotty baking.

Solution: Rotate the cookie sheet. Besides throwing out your oven, the next best thing to do to avoid hot spots is to rotate cookie sheets during baking. Turn cookie sheet around halfway through baking time to ensure even browning, especially for thin, roll-out, light-colored cookies. But do it quickly! Have your oven mitts on and act fast so that the oven doesn't cool down. Close that oven door as soon as you can, what were you, brought up in a barn?

Suspect #2: Dark baking sheet. Dark metal traps the heat while light metal reflects it. Don't blame us, blame science.

Solution: You might also want to switch over to light metal cookie sheets if you're using dark ones.

EXHIBIT E: *They're floppy and doughy*

Suspect: Your oven. Could be your cookies are underbaked. Do they appear pale and anemic? Do they have absolutely no browning on the bottom?

Solution: There's no saving this batch (unless you've just pulled them out of the oven, in which case stop reading this and get them back in!) but just bake the next batch a little longer. And, hey, have we mentioned that you need an oven thermometer (see page 25)? Because maybe you're baking at the wrong temp.

EXHIBIT F: *Rock-hard pucks*

Suspect: We're pretty sure by this point you have an oven thermometer, so it's not that your oven temperature is off kilter, is it?

Solution: Rock-hard texture usually means the cookies are overbaked. Check out "The Science of Cookies" (page 25) to make sure that this travesty never happens again.

EXHIBIT G: *Greasy grossness*

Suspect: Too much oil (obviously). So the cookie looks fine but seems to be leaving a trail of grease in its wake.

Solution: We're still not exactly sure why this happens. The obvious culprit is mismeasuring, but if you swear up and down you have measured correctly, we would suggest just cutting down the oil or margarine in the recipe the next time you make it. Remove around 2 tablespoons and see if that doesn't fix things for you.

PART TWO

THE RECIPES

DROP COOKIES

MIX IT, DROP IT, BAKE IT. Sometimes you gotta roll 'em into a ball or press 'em down, but no biggie—no other cookie satisfies as quickly and simply. Last-minute guests or on-the-spot cravings all respond to these free-form, minimal-equipment-required cookies. From the basics (chocolate chips and oatmeal) to the unexpected (cherries, pretzels, or macadamia nuts), we have a drop cookie for every demanding cookie fan in your life. So easy for even the busiest of bees, why not make a few different varieties whenever the need for cookies comes a knockin'?

CHOCOLATE CHIP COOKIES

MAKES 2 DOZEN 2-INCH COOKIES OR ABOUT 16 3-INCH COOKIES

THIS IS THE CHOCOLATE CHIP COOKIE that makes you feel like home. They're crinkly on the top, a little crispy on the bottom, and soft in the center. As an added bonus to the recipe, you only need one bowl for mixing the ingredients. Great for those of you in the no-dishwasher set.

½ cup brown sugar
¼ cup white sugar
⅔ cup canola oil
¼ cup unsweetened almond milk
   (or your favorite nondairy milk)
1 tablespoon tapioca flour
2 teaspoons pure vanilla extract
1½ cups all-purpose flour
½ teaspoon baking soda
½ teaspoon salt
¾ cup chocolate chips

1. Preheat oven to 350°F. Lightly grease two large baking sheets.
2. Combine sugars, oil, almond milk, and tapioca flour in a mixing bowl. Use a strong fork and mix really well, for about 2 minutes, until the mixture resembles smooth cara-mel. There is a chemical reaction when sugar and oil collide, so it's important that you don't get lazy about that step. Mix in the vanilla.
3. Add 1 cup of the flour, the baking soda, and the salt. Mix until well incorporated. Mix in the rest of the flour. Fold in the chocolate chips. The dough will be a little stiff so use your hands to really work the chips in.
4. For 3-inch cookies, roll the dough into balls about the size of Ping-Pong balls. Flatten them out in your hands to about 2½ inches. As they cook, they will spread just a bit. Place on a baking sheet and bake for about 8 minutes—no more than

9—until they are just a little browned around the edges. We usually get 16 out of these so we do two rounds of eight cookies. Let cool on the baking sheet for about 5 minutes then transfer to wire racks.

5. For two dozen 2-inch cookies roll dough into walnut-size balls and flatten to about 1½ inches and bake for only 6 minutes.

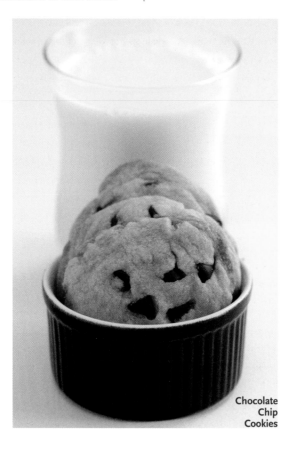

Chocolate
Chip
Cookies

VEGAN COOKIES INVADE YOUR COOKIE JAR

CARROT RAISIN SPICE CHEWIES

CARROT CAKE IN A COOKIE FORM, perfect for lunch boxes or mid-blogging snacking. These sweet treats are best eaten the day they're made, when the edges are crisp and the centers are soft. After that, they'll get chewy and moist all over, but still yum. Enjoy them naked, fancied up with a light drizzle of Lemon Glaze, or even smooshed together with a little vanilla dairy-free ice cream. These are easy enough to make healthier by substituting half whole wheat pastry flour for the all-purpose.

⅓ cup nondairy milk
1 tablespoon ground flax seeds
½ cup canola or peanut oil
⅓ cup dark brown sugar
1 cup sugar
½ teaspoon finely shredded orange zest
1½ teaspoons pure vanilla extract
1¾ cups all-purpose flour
1 teaspoon baking powder
1½ teaspoons ground cinnamon
1 teaspoon ground ginger
½ teaspoon ground nutmeg
½ teaspoon salt
1 cup finely shredded carrots, lightly packed
½ cup shredded coconut
½ cup chopped walnuts
1 cup raisins
LEMON GLAZE (page 38)

1. Preheat oven to 350°F. Generously grease two baking sheets or line them with parchment paper.
2. In a large bowl, beat together the nondairy milk, flax seeds, oil, brown sugar, sugar, orange zest, and vanilla. Sift in the flour, baking powder, cinnamon, ginger, nutmeg, and salt. Stir to moisten ingredients and fold in the carrots, coconut, walnuts, and raisins. Dough will be sticky and moist.
3. Drop generous tablespoons of dough onto cookie sheets, leaving about 2 inches of space between each. Bake for 14 to 16 minutes until the edges are brown and the tops

are firm. Let the cookies rest on the baking sheet for 10 minutes then transfer to wire racks to complete cooling.

Morsels

For best texture, use the smallest hole on your shredder to grate the carrots.

★ ★ ★

LEMON GLAZE

A quick and light drizzle to fancy up GINGERBREAD BISCOTTI (page 207) or any cookie.

1½ cups sifted powdered sugar
2 tablespoons lemon juice
½ teaspoon finely grated lemon zest

1. In a mixing bowl, whisk together all the ingredients using a fork or a wire whisk until smooth. Combine to form a glaze that's thin enough to drizzle from a fork or be easily piped from a pastry bag with a small round tip.
2. If the glaze is too thick, whisk in 1 teaspoon at a time of either nondairy milk or water. If it's too thin, whisk in more powdered sugar by the tablespoon until a desired consistency is reached.

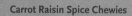
Carrot Raisin Spice Chewies

CHOCOLATE FUDGY OATMEAL COOKIES

MAKES 2-1/2 DOZEN COOKIES

ADD OATMEAL TO ALMOST ANYTHING and suddenly it's healthy! These cookies are chocolaty and fudgy, yet seem a perfectly acceptable afternoon pick-me-up with a dose of everybody's favorite whole grain. Dried cherries or raisins give them a grown-up touch, but if you're serving dried-fruit-a-phobes, they're just as good without.

2 cups quick-cooking oats
1⅔ cups all-purpose flour
⅔ cup cocoa powder
½ teaspoon baking soda
½ teaspoon baking powder
¾ teaspoon salt
1½ cups sugar
2 tablespoons ground flax seeds
⅔ cup nondairy milk
⅔ cup canola oil
1½ teaspoons pure vanilla extract
¼ teaspoon almond extract
¾ cup chocolate chips
1 cup dried cherries, chopped, or raisins
(optional)

1. Preheat oven to 350°F. Line two baking sheets with parchment paper.

2. In a medium-size bowl, stir together oats, flour, cocoa powder, baking soda, baking powder, and salt. Set aside.

3. In a large bowl, beat together sugar, flax seeds, and nondairy milk until smooth. Add the oil and the vanilla and almond extracts and beat until well mixed. Fold in half of the flour mixture to moisten, then fold in the remaining half. Just before the mixture is completely combined, fold in the chocolate chips and dried cherries or raisins, if desired.

4. For each cookie drop 2 generous tablespoons of dough onto the cookie sheet, leaving about 2 inches of space between each cookie. If

desired, flatten slightly with moistened fingers or the moistened back of a measuring cup. Bake for 10 to 12 minutes until cookies are firm and risen. Let the cookies rest on the baking sheet for 5 minutes then transfer to wire racks to complete cooling. Store in a tightly covered container.

Morsels

Leave the dough unflattened for more chewy cookies or flatten a bit for a firmer texture.

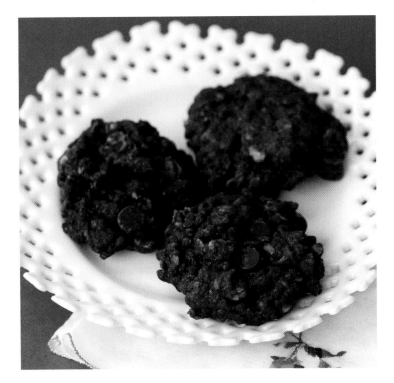

BLACKSTRAP GINGERSNAPS

MAKES ABOUT 2 DOZEN COOKIES

WHEN ONLY AN ASSERTIVELY GINGER cookie will do. These are not the soft type of molasses cookie, rather they are firm and crisp when freshly baked, developing a chewy finish the next day or in humid weather. One could consider these "snappy," perhaps. The rich and slightly bitter-tasting blackstrap variety is the molasses of choice for this cookie, but regular molasses can be substituted as well.

¾ cup sugar
⅓ cup blackstrap molasses
½ cup canola oil
3 tablespoons nondairy milk
½ teaspoon pure vanilla extract
1¾ cups all-purpose flour, or use half all-purpose and half whole wheat pastry
3 rounded teaspoons ground ginger
½ teaspoon ground nutmeg
½ teaspoon baking soda
½ teaspoon salt

1. Preheat oven to 350°F. Lightly grease two baking sheets or line them with parchment paper.

2. In a large bowl, beat together sugar, molasses, oil, nondairy milk, and vanilla. In a separate bowl sift together flour, ginger, nutmeg, baking soda, and salt. Fold the dry mixture into the wet to form a firm dough.

3. Scoop dough by the tablespoon, moisten hands, and roll into a ball. Place dough balls about 3 inches apart on baking sheets, and flatten slightly. Bake for 12 minutes until edges start to brown. Let the cookies rest on the baking sheet for 5 minutes, then transfer to wire racks to complete cooling. Store in a loosely covered container.

CHOCOLATY CRINKLE COOKIES

POWDERED SUGAR REALLY SETS THE MOOD for holiday cookies. Here are those chocolaty, fudgy-centered wonders with the dramatic contrasting of dark crinkles and the snowy sweet stuff. These cookies look best when served the day of baking but will still be as tasty as ever the next day. Black cocoa provides the sharpest-looking cocoa, but use regular cocoa powder if that's all you've got.

FOR ROLLING COOKIES:
   1½ cups powdered sugar
   ⅓ cup sugar

FOR THE DOUGH:
   ¾ cup sugar
   ⅓ cup canola oil
   2 tablespoons dark corn syrup
   1 teaspoon pure vanilla extract
   ⅓ cup nondairy milk
   1 tablespoon ground flax seeds
   4 ounces (about ½ cup) chocolate
      chips, melted
   1¼ cups plus 2 tablespoons all-purpose
      flour
   2 tablespoons black cocoa powder or
      natural cocoa powder
   ¾ teaspoon baking powder
   ¼ teaspoon salt

1. Preheat oven to 325°F. Line two baking sheets with parchment paper.
2. Sift the powdered sugar that will be used for rolling the cookies onto a large plate, preferably one with a raised edge. Pour the sugar for rolling into a small separate bowl. Set these aside.
3. In a large bowl, mix together sugar, oil, corn syrup, vanilla, nondairy milk, flax seeds, and melted chocolate until smooth. Sift in flour, black cocoa powder, baking powder, and salt and mix until a moist, thick dough forms. You can bake it

Chocolaty Crinkle Cookies

as is, or for easier handling of dough, chill it for 15 to 20 minutes.

4. For each cookie, scoop a generous tablespoon of dough and roll it into a ball. First roll the ball in the sugar, then roll several times in the powdered sugar. Don't be stingy with rolling in both the granulated and powdered sugars; the more powdered sugar each cookie is coated with, the prettier it will look after it's baked.

5. Place balls of dough at least 2 inches apart on lined baking sheets, as these will spread. Bake for 14 minutes until cookies are puffed and cracks have formed on the surface. Remove the cookies from the oven and let them cool on the baking sheet for at least 5 minutes, then use a thin spatula to carefully move them to wire racks to finish cooling. Store in a tightly covered container.

Morsels

This is perhaps the only recipe in this book that calls for corn syrup, if just a few tablespoons of it. However, it really does give these cookies exceptional spreading power and helps form the pretty cracks. If you're not ready to commit to this hot-button sweetener, many of our testers had success substituting brown rice syrup. The results look pretty good, but may not have as much spread as the cookies shown.

CITY GIRL SNICKERDOODLES

WE ARE GOING TO MAKE A CONFESSION: we really don't know the classic Pennsylvania Dutch snickerdoodle very well. So snickerdoodle veterans out there, consider these a variation for us city folk. They don't seem to be much of a presence in the Northeast, which is a shame because this cookie just radiates yumminess that can stop traffic. This thin, crisp, buttery cookie coated in cinnamon sugar is pretty much perfect alone, but if necessary, serve with a little dairy-free vanilla ice cream. The addition of decorator sugar makes it just a little extra-glittery and girly.

1 cup nonhydrogenated margarine, softened
1¼ cups sugar
2 tablespoons nondairy milk
1½ teaspoons pure vanilla extract
1⅔ cups all-purpose flour
¼ cup cornstarch
1 teaspoon cream of tartar
½ teaspoon baking soda
¼ teaspoon salt

CINNAMON SUGAR FOR ROLLING:
⅓ cup sugar
2 tablespoons white decorator sugar, or any large-crystal sugar
1 rounded teaspoon ground cinnamon
A big pinch of ground nutmeg

1. In a large bowl cream the margarine and sugar together until light and creamy, about 3 minutes, scraping the sides of the bowl when necessary. Add the nondairy milk and vanilla and beat until combined. Sift in the flour, cornstarch, cream of tartar, baking soda, and salt and beat mixture until a soft dough forms, about 4 minutes. Dough will be soft and fluffy. Chill dough for 30 minutes. Or, if desired, cover the dough with plastic wrap and chill overnight.

2. Preheat oven to 350°F and line two baking sheets with parchment paper. In a small shallow bowl, combine the sugar, decorator sugar, cinnamon, and nutmeg.

3. Scoop 1 tablespoon of dough, drop it into Cinnamon Sugar, and gently roll it into a ball. Place dough balls on cookie sheets about 3 inches apart. Sprinkle the top of each cookie with a little additional Cinnamon Sugar.

4. Bake 10 to 12 minutes. Cookies will be puffed and will deflate after removing from the oven. Allow cookies to cool 5 minutes on the baking sheets before moving to wire racks to complete cooling. Store in a loosely covered container.

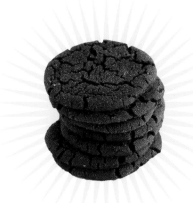

COWBOY COOKIES

MAKES 2 DOZEN LARGE COOKIES

WE'VE HEARD OF THIS LEGENDARY VARIETY of oatmeal cookie and really have no idea what makes it "cowboy," but we like it just the same. Can't you picture a big, mustached cowboy on the range just chowing down on these babies instead of nasty old beef jerky? But we digress. Here's our version of that big, satisfying oat and brown sugar cookie, chock full of all kinds of things like nuts, coconut, and best of all, chocolate. Vegan chocolate chunks are perfect for this cookie, so use them if you can find 'em!

2 cups quick-cooking oats
2 cups all-purpose flour
1 teaspoon baking soda
½ teaspoon baking powder
½ teaspoon salt
⅔ cup canola or peanut oil
⅔ cup sugar
¾ cup firmly packed dark brown sugar
½ cup nondairy milk
1 tablespoon ground flax seeds
1 teaspoon pure vanilla extract
1 cup shredded coconut
1 generous cup semisweet chocolate chunks or chips
1 cup chopped toasted pecan pieces
Additional nuts and chocolate chips or chunks for decorating tops of cookies.

1. Preheat oven to 350°F. Line two baking sheets with parchment paper.
2. In a medium-size bowl, stir together oats, flour, baking soda, baking powder, and salt. Set aside.
3. In a large bowl, beat together oil, sugar, brown sugar, nondairy milk, flax seeds, and vanilla. Fold in half of the flour mixture to moisten, then fold in the remaining half. Just before the mixture is completely combined, fold in the coconut, chocolate chunks, and pecans.
4. For each cookie, drop ¼ cup of dough (about the size of a golf ball)

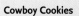

Cowboy Cookies

onto cookie sheets. The dough will be sticky and thick. Leave about 2 inches of space between each cookie. Flatten slightly with moistened fingers or the moistened back of a measuring cup; repeat dipping in water for each cookie. Bake for 14–16 minutes until edges start to brown. Let the cookies rest on the baking sheet for 5 minutes then transfer to wire racks to complete cooling. Store in a loosely covered container. These are also ideal cookie jar cookies!

Variation

COWGIRL COOKIES: Omit the coconut and pecans. With the flour, sift in 1½ teaspoons ground cinnamon and ¼ teaspoon ground cloves. At the end of the mixing process, stir in 1 cup dried cranberries, 1 cup toasted walnut pieces, and 1 generous cup semisweet chocolate chunks or chips *or* vegan white chocolate chips.

Morsels

A lazy way to toast pecans is to make use of that preheating oven, since nuts like to be toasted in low heat. Spread them on a cookie sheet and 5 minutes into turning the oven on, pop the sheet right in. Bake for 6 to 10 minutes, watching very carefully! Nuts should be fragrant and just barely browned. Remove the nuts from the oven and allow them to cool before chopping or breaking into smaller pieces, if necessary.

SELL YOUR SOUL PUMPKIN COOKIES

MAKES 2 DOZEN COOKIES

PUMPKIN COOKIES ARE USUALLY kind of fluffy and cakey, which is nice, but we wanted something with a firmer, more cookie-like bite. To accomplish this, we could either sell our souls or cook the pumpkin down to reduce the moisture content. We did both for good measure. You need to cook the pumpkin down for about 45 minutes, so keep that in mind for cookie time management purposes.

1 cup canned pumpkin
½ cup nonhydrogenated vegetable shortening
½ cup sugar
½ cup packed brown sugar
1 teaspoon pure vanilla extract
1½ cups all-purpose flour
¼ cup oat flour (make your own by whirring rolled oats in a food processor)
2 tablespoons cornstarch
1½ teaspoons ground cinnamon
1 teaspoon ground ginger
½ teaspoon ground nutmeg
¼ teaspoon ground cloves
½ teaspoon baking powder
½ teaspoon salt
A handful of shelled pumpkin seeds for garnish (optional)

1. First, reduce the pumpkin. Place it in a saucepan over medium heat for about 45 minutes. Keep the heat low enough that it doesn't boil, but it should appear to be steaming. Stir often. After about 30 minutes, spoon the pumpkin into a liquid measuring cup to check on how much it has reduced. It should be down to around ⅔ cup at this point. Return the pumpkin to pot to cook until it has reduced to ½ cup. Set aside to cool completely.

2. Preheat oven to 350°F. Line two baking sheets with parchment paper.

3. In a large mixing bowl, use a hand mixer to cream together the shortening and sugars until light and fluffy. Mix in the cooled pumpkin and vanilla.

4. Sift in all remaining ingredients and mix to combine. Spoon onto cookie sheets in rounded tablespoons of dough, flattening the tops with your hand. Arrange a few pumpkin seeds in the centers, if you like.

5. Bake for 10 to 12 minutes. Remove the cookies from the oven and let them cool on the cookie sheet for 5 minutes. Transfer the cookies to wire racks to cool completely.

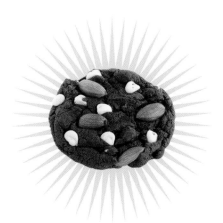

Sell Your Soul Pumpkin Cookies

Espresso Chip Oatmeal Cookies

Morsels

Look for instant Italian espresso powder at gourmet markets in the coffee aisle or even in the baking aisles at fancy supermarkets. Instant espresso powder has a rich, concentrated flavor that's magical in baked goods. If you can't find it, it's okay to substitute instant coffee granules; the flavor will just not be as intense.

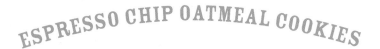

ESPRESSO CHIP OATMEAL COOKIES

MAKES 2 DOZEN COOKIES

OATMEAL COOKIES WITH A DASH OF ESPRESSO and a thoughtful helping of chocolate chips will bring a little extra vroom-vroom to your afternoon snacking. Rumored to be an excellent, if occasional, addition to mornings on-the-go-go, too.

½ cup nondairy milk
½ cup canola oil
2 tablespoons ground flax seeds
⅓ cup brown sugar
½ cup sugar
1 teaspoon pure vanilla extract
⅔ cups all-purpose flour
⅛ teaspoon ground cinnamon
2 tablespoons instant espresso powder
1 tablespoon cocoa powder
¾ teaspoon baking powder
¼ teaspoon salt
1¾ cups quick-cooking oats
¾ cup chocolate chips

1. Preheat oven to 350°F. Line two baking sheets with parchment paper.
2. In a large bowl, mix together nondairy milk, oil, flax seeds, brown sugar, sugar, and vanilla until smooth. Sift in flour, cinnamon, espresso powder, cocoa powder, baking powder, and salt. Add quick-cooking oats and chocolate chips and stir until all ingredients are moistened.
3. Drop generous tablespoons of dough about 2 inches apart onto baking sheets. Bake for 14 minutes, until cookies are slightly puffed and the edges appear dry.
4. Let the cookies cool on baking sheets for 5 minutes, then transfer them to wire racks to cool completely. Store in a loosely covered container.

Morsels
Substitute more
vanilla extract if
there's no coconut
to be had.

Macadamia Ginger Crunch Drops

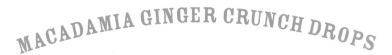

MACADAMIA GINGER CRUNCH DROPS

MAKES 2-1/2 DOZEN COOKIES

CANDIED GINGER FANS GET THEIR DAY with these morsels. Rich, sweet, and subtly spicy, these cookies also pack a big huge crunch with plenty of tasty macs. Dreamy indeed with a cup of chai.

2 cups all-purpose flour
½ teaspoon baking soda
½ teaspoon salt
¼ teaspoon ground nutmeg
⅔ cup canola oil
⅔ cup sugar
¾ cup firmly packed dark brown sugar
⅓ cup nondairy milk
1 tablespoon ground flax seeds
1½ teaspoons pure vanilla extract
½ teaspoon coconut extract
6 ounces (about 1⅓ cups) unsalted macadamia nuts, chopped
4 ounces (about ½ generous cup) candied ginger, finely chopped

1. Preheat oven to 350°F. Line two baking sheets with parchment paper.
2. In a medium-size bowl, sift together flour, baking soda, salt, and nutmeg.
3. In a large bowl, beat together oil, sugar, brown sugar, nondairy milk, flax seeds, and the vanilla and coconut extracts. Fold in the flour mixture and mix to moisten. Just before mixture is completely combined, fold in the macadamia nuts and ginger.
4. For each cookie, drop 1 generous tablespoon of dough onto the cookie sheet. The dough will be sticky and thick. Leave about 2 inches of space between each cookie.
5. Bake for 14 minutes until edges start to brown. Let the cookies rest on baking sheet for 5 minutes, then transfer them to wire racks to complete cooling. Store in a tightly covered container.

BANANA EVERYTHING COOKIES

MAKES 2 DOZEN COOKIES

BANANA AND WALNUTS ARE BEST BUDS in this chewy cookie. It's a clean-out-your-cupboard kind of cookie, unless you don't have any of the ingredients, in which case it's a go-to-the-grocery-store cookie.

1 very ripe medium banana
⅓ cup canola oil
⅔ cup sugar
1 teaspoon vanilla
¾ cup plus 2 tablespoons all-purpose flour
½ teaspoon baking soda
¼ teaspoon salt
¼ teaspoon ground cinnamon
2 cups quick-cooking (*not* instant) oatmeal or rolled oats
½ cup chopped walnuts
½ cup chocolate chips

1. Preheat oven to 350°F. Lightly grease two baking sheets.
2. In a mixing bowl, mash the banana well. You can use a fork for this, but your hands work well, too. Add the oil, sugar, and vanilla and mix with a strong fork. Add the flour, baking soda, salt, and cinnamon and mix until the dry ingredients are just moistened. Add the oatmeal, walnuts, and chocolate chips and mix well. It's actually good to use your hands for mixing when using oatmeal, that way you make sure that the oats get nice and moist. If the dough is very slippery you might want to add a few tablespoons extra flour—it really depends on how big your banana was.
3. Clean your hands and roll the dough into balls slightly smaller than a golf ball. Flatten it a bit in your hands and place each ball

58 VEGAN COOKIES INVADE YOUR COOKIE JAR

about 2 inches apart on the cookie sheet.

4. Bake for 10 to 12 minutes, until lightly browned. Let the cookies cool on the cookie sheet for 2 minutes, then transfer them to a cooling rack.

Variation

BREKKY BANANA COOKIES: This also makes a great breakfast cookie if you omit the chocolate chips and add 2 tablespoons of ground flax seeds to the flour.

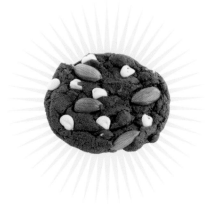

TAHINI LIME COOKIES

MAKES 2 DOZEN COOKIES

REMINISCENT OF SESAME HALVAH, tahini gives these cookies a sultry and almost mysterious taste. Flecks of lime zest brighten them up and a sprinkle of black sesame seeds on top lets you know what's what. Because tahinis have varying oil content, you may have to add a little extra nondairy milk if the dough appears too dry.

½ cup nonhydrogenated vegetable shortening, softened
¾ cup sugar
½ cup tahini, at room temperature
3 to 5 tablespoons nondairy milk
Grated zest from two limes (about 1 tablespoon)
1 teaspoon pure vanilla extract
1¼ cups flour
2 tablespoons cornstarch
½ teaspoon baking powder
½ teaspoon salt
¼ cup black sesame seeds

1. Preheat oven to 350°F. Line two large baking sheets with parchment paper.
2. In a large mixing bowl, use a hand mixer at medium speed to beat together the shortening and sugar until light and fluffy. Beat in the tahini, 3 tablespoons of the nondairy milk, and the zest. Mix in the vanilla.
3. Add half the flour along with the cornstarch, baking powder, and salt and mix well. Add the remaining flour and mix. Use your hands at this point to really work the ingredients together. The dough should hold together when squeezed; if it does not then add a tablespoon or two of nondairy milk until it does.
4. Roll dough into walnut-size balls and flatten them a bit with the palms of your hand. The dough may crack on the edges and that is

fine. Place the dough balls on the cookie sheets and flatten them a little bit more. Sprinkle and lightly press sesame seeds into the tops.

5. Bake for 10 to 12 minutes, until the edges are very lightly browned. Remove the cookies from the oven and let them cool on the sheets for 10 minutes. Use a thin, flexible spatula to transfer them to a rack to cool completely.

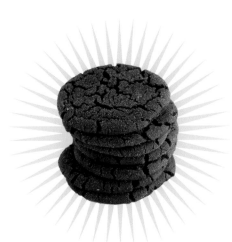

Cherry Almond Cookies

CHERRY ALMOND COOKIES

CHERRIES AND ALMONDS ARE ALWAYS SIMPATICO, and this cookie is no exception. The cherries turn these cookies into pretty little jewels, so don't be surprised if your cookie jar gets robbed in the middle of the night.

⅓ cup canola oil
⅓ cup sugar
⅓ cup firmly packed brown sugar
3 tablespoons nondairy milk
2 teaspoons ground flax seeds
1 teaspoon pure vanilla extract
½ teaspoon almond extract
1 cup all-purpose flour
¼ teaspoon baking soda
¼ teaspoon salt
¾ cup slivered almonds
¾ cup dried cherries

1. Preheat oven to 350°F. Line two medium-size baking sheets with parchment paper.

2. In a large bowl, use a fork to vigorously mix oil, sugars, nondairy milk, flax seeds, and extracts. Sift in flour, baking soda, and salt and mix. When ingredients are mostly combined, add the almonds and cherries and mix until thoroughly combined.

3. Drop cookies by generous tablespoons onto the baking sheets, about 2 inches apart. Bake for 10 to 12 minutes, until the edges begin to brown. Let the cookies rest on the baking sheet for 5 minutes before transferring them to wire racks to complete cooling.

PEANUT APPLE PRETZEL DROPS

MAKES OVER 2-1/2 DOZEN COOKIES

OUR FRIEND EVELYN TOLD US that she loves to snack on the sweet 'n' salty combo of pretzels and apples, and we made it even better by adding peanuts. A delicate brown sugar cookie dough brings this trio of awesome together for a perfectly chewy yet crunchy delight, sure to thrill young, old, or simply those who like to act immature. Enjoy as a wholesome after-school or post-work snack with a cold glass of soy milk. (Note: with all the chunky mix-ins, these cookies will look a little crazy. Don't be scared if they appear a little more free-form than you're used to.)

2 generous cups mini pretzels, crushed into small pieces
1 cup roasted, shelled peanut halves
4 ounces (about 1½ cups, lightly packed) dried apple rings
1¾ cups flour
½ teaspoon baking powder
½ teaspoon baking soda
¼ teaspoon ground cinnamon
¼ teaspoon salt
½ cup nondairy milk
2 tablespoons ground flax seeds
½ cup canola oil
1 cup dark brown sugar, tightly packed
⅓ cup sugar
1½ teaspoons pure vanilla extract

1. Preheat oven to 350°F. Line two baking sheets with parchment paper.

2. In a large bowl, combine pretzel pieces and peanuts. Using either kitchen scissors or a sharp knife, cut apple rings into bite-size pieces. Combine with the pretzels and peanuts.

3. In a large mixing bowl, sift together the flour, baking powder, baking soda, cinnamon, and salt.

4. In a separate large bowl, whisk together the nondairy milk and flax seeds. Add the oil, brown sugar, sugar, and vanilla. Beat with elec-

Peanut Apple Pretzel Drops

tric beaters for 2 minutes until the lumps of brown sugar are dissolved and the mixture is very thick. Stir in the flour mixture, mixing just until dry ingredients are moistened and a thick, soft dough forms (you might want to use a rubber spatula for this step). Fold in the pretzel mixture and stir to completely coat everything with batter. The result-

ing dough will be very chunky and sticky.

5. Drop heaping tablespoons of dough about 2 inches apart onto the baking sheet. Bake 14 to 16 minutes until cookies are firm and edges are lightly browned. Move from the cookie sheet to wire racks to cool. Store in a loosely covered container.

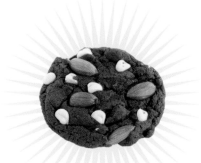

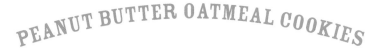

PEANUT BUTTER OATMEAL COOKIES

PEANUT BUTTER AND OATMEAL PARTNER UP to create another stick-to-your-ribs oatmeal cookie, even wholesome enough for breakfast if you must eat cookies then. Briefly rolling the dough in salted peanuts really makes this one, so definitely use those over the unsalted variety. For serious ice cream sandwiches, serve this excellent cookie with vanilla chocolate chip dairy-free ice cream.

1⅓ cups all-purpose flour, or a combination of whole wheat pastry and all-purpose
1 teaspoon baking powder
¾ teaspoon baking soda
1¼ teaspoons ground cinnamon
½ teaspoon salt
2 cups oats, quick-cooking or rolled
½ cup canola oil
½ cup creamy natural peanut butter
½ cup sugar
¾ cup firmly packed dark brown sugar
⅓ cup nondairy milk
4 teaspoons ground flax seeds
1½ teaspoons pure vanilla extract
1 cup roasted, salted peanuts, chopped

1. Preheat oven to 350°F. Lightly grease two baking sheets or line them with parchment paper.

2. In a medium-size bowl, sift together flour, baking powder, baking soda, cinnamon, and salt. Stir in the oats and set aside.

3. In a large bowl, beat together oil, peanut butter, sugar, brown sugar, nondairy milk, flax seeds, and vanilla until smooth. Fold in half of the flour/oat mixture to moisten, then fold in the remaining half.

4. Place the chopped salted peanuts in a shallow dish. Drop 1 generous, rounded tablespoon of dough per cookie into the peanuts, pressing

Peanut Butter Oatmeal Cookies

the nuts into the dough. Move the dough onto the cookie sheets, leaving about 2 inches of space between each cookie. Flatten slightly with moistened fingers or the moistened back of a measuring cup.

5. Bake for 12 to 14 minutes until the edges just start to brown. Let the cookies rest on the baking sheet for 5 minutes before transferring to wire racks to complete cooling. Store loosely covered.

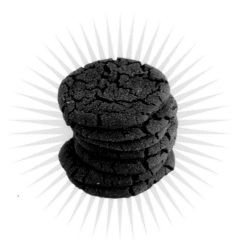

CITRUS GLITTERS

A SOFT CITRUS COOKIE ENCASED IN A GLITTERY SHELL, thanks to a dip in turbinado sugar. This cookie is a true miracle worker, managing to be round and fluffy without being too cakey. We used a mix of orange, lemon, and lime zest, but really you can use whatever citrus you have lying around.

3 to 4 tablespoons turbinado, demerara, or other coarse sugar
½ cup nonhydrogenated vegetable shortening, softened
¾ cup sugar
¼ cup almond milk
2 tablespoons finely grated citrus zest (from oranges, lemons, and limes)
1 teaspoon pure vanilla extract
1¾ cups all-purpose flour
2 tablespoons fine-ground cornmeal (see tip)
1 tablespoon cornstarch
½ teaspoon baking powder
¼ teaspoon salt

1. Preheat oven to 350°F. Line two baking sheets with parchment paper. Spoon the turbinado sugar onto a plate and set aside.

2. Use a hand mixer at medium speed to cream the shortening and granulated sugar until light and fluffy, about a minute and a half. Mix in the almond milk, citrus zest, and vanilla.

3. Add all remaining ingredients and mix on medium speed until a soft, pliable dough forms. It might look crumbly, but when pressed between your fingers it should come together easily.

4. Roll heaping tablespoons of dough into balls. Press each ball into the turbinado sugar to flatten it into a tire shape, coating one side only. Place the cookies, sugar side up, on the baking sheets. Bake for 10 to

12 minutes, until lightly golden around the edges. Let the cookies cool on the baking sheets for 2 minutes, then transfer them to wire racks to cool completely. Store in a tightly sealed container.

Morsels

If your cornmeal is medium or coarse ground, give it a whirl in the food processor.

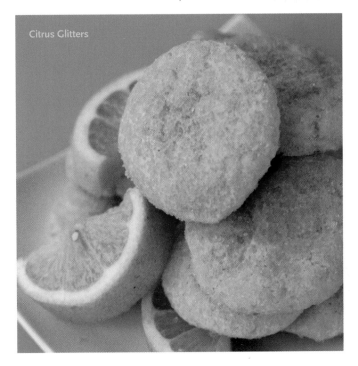

Citrus Glitters

Pignoli Almond Cookies

PIGNOLI ALMOND COOKIES

MAKES 2 DOZEN COOKIES

RICH, BUTTERY ALMOND FLAVOR, a dense chewy center, and a sprinkle of pine nuts make these Italian bakery–inspired cookies special. Pignoli cookies are holiday favorites, too, so include a batch at your next big-time cookie swap. Make sure to use only almond paste and not marzipan here; we like the almond paste that comes in a handy foil-wrapped tube, but any kind will do the trick.

7 ounces almond paste, sliced into
    1-inch cubes
A pinch of salt
½ teaspoon baking powder
⅔ cup sugar
½ cup nonhydrogenated margarine,
    softened
½ teaspoon almond extract
1 cup all-purpose flour
½ cup pine nuts
2 to 3 tablespoons almond milk for
    dipping

1. Preheat oven to 325°F. Line two medium-size baking sheets with parchment paper.

2. Pulse almond paste, salt, baking powder, and ⅓ cup of the sugar in a food processor until mixture is crumbly, about 1 minute.

3. In a large bowl, cream together the margarine and remaining ⅓ cup sugar with an electric mixer until mixture is pale and fluffy, about 3 minutes. Add the almond paste mixture and almond extract and beat until fluffy, about 2 minutes. Sift in the flour and beat until a slightly crumbly yet soft dough forms.

4. Pour the pine nuts into a shallow bowl and pour 2 tablespoons of almond milk into a small saucer. For each cookie scoop 1 tablespoon of dough and roll it in your palms to

form into a ball. Dip one end of the ball in the almond milk and press this moistened end into pine nuts. If necessary, use your fingers to press the pine nuts into the dough. Place the dough balls, pine nut side up, on a baking sheet at least 2 inches apart. Bake for 14 minutes until cookies have puffed and spread a little and the nuts are just slightly toasted. Remove from the oven and allow the cookies to cool on the baking sheet for 5 minutes to firm up before carefully transferring them to wire racks. Store in a tightly covered container.

Morsels

These cookies are super-soft right out of the oven, so be sure to allow them a full 5 minutes to firm up on the cookie sheet before transferring to wire racks to complete cooling.

OATMEAL RAISIN COOKIES

MAKES 2 DOZEN COOKIES

NO ONE REALLY KNOWS WHERE OR HOW these humble ingredients came together to form the power couple of the cookie world, but we'll just have to chalk it up as one of life's happy little miracles. Some people prefer a chewy oatmeal raisin cookie and some prefer crunchy, so here's a little secret: 10 minutes in the oven will get you your chewy cookies and 12 minutes will get you your crunchies.

⅓ cup soy milk
2 tablespoons ground flax seeds
⅔ cup brown sugar
⅓ cup oil
1 teaspoon pure vanilla extract
¾ cup flour
½ teaspoon ground cinnamon
⅛ teaspoon ground nutmeg
¼ teaspoon baking soda
¼ teaspoon salt
1½ cups quick-cooking oats
½ cup raisins

1. Preheat oven to 350°F. Line two baking sheets with parchment paper.

2. In a large bowl, use a fork to vigorously mix together the soy milk and flax seeds. Add in the sugar and oil and mix until it resembles caramel, about 2 minutes. Mix in the vanilla. Sift in the flour, spices, and salt, mixing the dry ingredients as they are being added. Fold in the oatmeal and raisins.

3. Drop dough in generous tablespoons, about 2 inches apart, onto the baking sheets. Flatten the tops a bit, since they don't spread much. Bake for 10 to 12 minutes.

4. Let cool on the baking sheets for 5 minutes, then transfer to wire racks to cool completely. Store in a tightly covered container.

Morsels

If your raisins are looking a little under the weather, a tad too dry or sticking together, place them in a bowl and pour warm water over them. This will plump them up and bring them back to life.

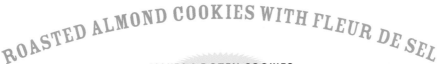

ROASTED ALMOND COOKIES WITH FLEUR DE SEL

MAKES 2 DOZEN COOKIES

PRESENTING A DIFFERENT SET OF COOKIE FLAVORS: just a hint of sweetness, deep roasted almonds, caramel-like brown rice syrup, and a sprinkling of *fleur de sel* to top it off. Think of these as a slightly savory vacation from super-sweet treats, almost adult-tasting, if you will. The spices are kept simple here to let the flavor of the almonds, salt, and rolled oats shine. Here's the recipe to bring out that fancy, large-grain salt of any kind; even flaky kosher salt will do in a pinch.

½ cup canola oil
⅓ cup brown rice syrup
⅔ cup dark brown sugar
⅓ cup nondairy milk
1 teaspoon vanilla extract
1 cup all-purpose flour
⅔ cup whole wheat pastry flour
1 teaspoon baking soda
½ teaspoon ground cinnamon
¼ teaspoon salt
1 cup roasted whole almonds, measured
    first then roughly chopped
1½ cups rolled oats
1 teaspoon or less of *fleur de sel* or any
    coarse-grained salt, for sprinkling

1. Preheat oven to 350°F. Line two medium-size baking sheets with parchment paper.

2. In a large bowl, mix together the oil, brown rice syrup, brown sugar, nondairy milk, and vanilla until smooth. Sift in the all-purpose flour, whole wheat pastry flour, baking soda, cinnamon, and salt and stir to moisten ingredients. Fold in the almonds and rolled oats. The batter will appear rather wet but will firm up a bit within a few minutes.

3. Drop dough in generous table-spoons, about 2 inches apart, onto the baking sheet. Lightly sprinkle

the tops of the cookies with coarse-grained salt. Bake for 10 to 12 minutes, until the cookies are slightly puffed and the edges appear dry.

4. Let cool on the baking sheet for 5 minutes, then transfer to wire racks to cool completely. Store in a loosely covered container as these cookies get soft if tightly covered.

✳ *Morsels* ✳

✦ A cookie warning, so pay attention! Go very easy on the salt when sprinkling the tops of these cookies. Six to eight large grains of salt may suffice, unless a bouillon cube cookie sounds good to you.

✦ For best flavor and appearance, use whole roasted almonds with the brown skin still on.

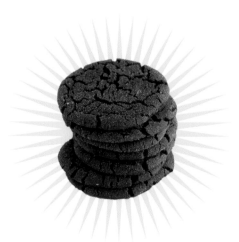

ROCKY ROADS

THE CLASSIC ICE CREAM FLAVOR in a portable form that doesn't require a freezer or cone. A chewy, crispy, chocolaty cookie enrobes chips of both the chocolate and white chocolate persuasion, plus chunks of roasted almonds. A fun drop cookie when you're feeling that more is more! Definitely a nondairy milk 'n' cookies kind of cookie and a no-brainer for filling up the cookie jar.

This cookie dough is rather wet, so don't be alarmed and just trust us. Just scoop away and leave plenty of room between blobs of dough for spreading. If the wet dough freaks you out too much, place the entire bowl in the fridge for 30 minutes to firm up, keeping the bowl of dough chilled in between baking up batches.

½ cup nondairy milk
2 tablespoons ground flax seeds
½ cup canola oil
1¼ cups sugar
2 teaspoons vanilla extract
½ teaspoon almond extract
1½ cups plus 2 tablespoons all-purpose flour
½ cup Dutch cocoa powder
½ teaspoon baking soda
¼ teaspoon baking powder
½ teaspoon salt
½ cup chocolate chips or chunks
½ cup vegan white chocolate chips
½ cup roasted almonds, chopped

1. Preheat oven to 350°F. Line two baking sheets with parchment paper.

2. In a large mixing bowl, combine nondairy milk, flax seeds, oil, sugar, vanilla extract, and almond extract. Mix until well blended and smooth. Sift in all-purpose flour, cocoa powder, baking soda, baking powder, and salt. Stir to form a thick, wet dough but do not overmix. Fold in chocolate chips, white chocolate chips, and almonds. If

the dough seems too sticky, chill for 30 minutes to firm up, but this step is not essential.

3. For each cookie, drop about 2 tablespoons of dough onto a baking sheet 2 inches apart, as cookies will spread. Spray the spoon or dough scoop with nonstick spray if the dough is sticking.

4. Bake cookies for 8 to 10 minutes, until spread and cracked on top. Let the cookies cool on the baking sheet for 5 minutes, then transfer them to wire racks to cool completely. Store in a loosely covered container.

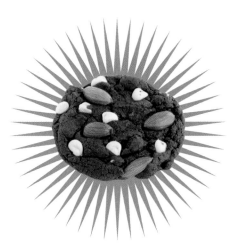

On cover (and above!): Rocky Roads Cookie.
Naturally gorgeous, no photo retouching necessary.

PEANUT BUTTER CRISSCROSSES

MAKES 2 DOZEN COOKIES

THE CLASSIC CROSS-HATCHED TOP in a light and delicate shortbread cookie. The idea here is to limit the amount of liquid you use, but because peanut butter moisture varies from brand to brand (and due to other mysterious cookie happenings), your dough might be dry. If it is then add a tablespoon or two of soy milk to the dough, but try without it at first because the tenderness of the cookie without the additional liquid is such a gosh darn delight.

½ cup nonhydrogenated vegetable shortening

½ cup natural smooth peanut butter (try to get the no-stir kind if you can find it. If you can't, then stir like crazy so that the PB isn't clumpy).

¾ cup sugar

1 teaspoon pure vanilla extract

2 tablespoons light molasses (not blackstrap)

1¼ cups flour

2 tablespoons cornstarch

½ teaspoon baking powder

½ teaspoon salt

1 to 2 tablespoons nondairy milk (optional)

1. Preheat oven to 350°F. Lightly grease two cookie sheets. We prefer dark cookie sheets here to get the cookies browned and crispy (see "Tools for Success," page 21).

2. In a large mixing bowl, beat together the shortening, peanut butter, and sugar until light and fluffy. This can take up to 2 minutes with an electric mixer at medium speed or 4 minutes just using a fork. Mix in the vanilla and molasses.

3. Add half the flour along with the cornstarch, baking powder, and salt and mix well. Add the remaining flour and mix. Use your hands at this point to really work the ingredients together. The dough should hold together when squeezed; if it

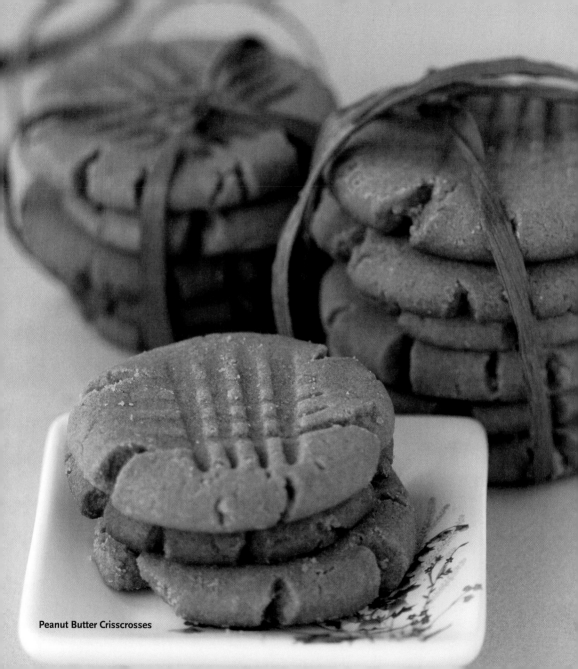

Peanut Butter Crisscrosses

does not, then add a tablespoon or two of nondairy milk until it does.

4. Roll the dough into walnut-size balls, flattening them a bit with the palms of your hand. The dough may crack on the edges and that is fine. Place the dough balls on the cookie sheets. Flatten them further with the bottom of a coffee mug. Use the underside of fork tines to press cross hatches into the cookies, one horizontal and one vertical.

5. Bake the cookies for 10 to 12 minutes, until the edges are very lightly browned. Remove the cookies from the oven and let them cool on the sheets for 10 minutes—any less and they might crumble. Use a thin, flexible spatula to transfer the cookies to wire racks to cool completely.

SWEET WINE BISCUITS WITH SESAME

MAKES ABOUT 3 DOZEN SMALL COOKIES

GROWN-UP COOKIE ALERT! These crisp, melt-in-your-mouth little guys deliver a surprising combo of sweet port wine, fruity olive oil, and just enough sweetness to balance out the savory sesame exterior. The port adds a rich afterthought that would be ideal served up with espresso. Or, make a big after-dinner deal about it paired with dessert wine, fresh fruit, and roasted cashews. Or even nibbled with little slices of your favorite faux cheese, if it pleases you.

½ cup sweet port wine
½ cup extra virgin olive oil
¾ cup sugar
½ teaspoon finely grated lemon zest
1⅔ cups all-purpose flour
½ teaspoon baking soda
½ teaspoon salt
⅔ cup white sesame seeds, for rolling

1. Preheat oven to 350°F. Line two medium-size baking sheets with parchment paper.

2. In a large bowl, whisk together port wine, oil, sugar, and lemon zest until thick. Sift in the flour, baking soda, and salt. Mix until the dry ingredients are completely moistened and a thick dough forms. The dough will be very sticky, so cover it with plastic wrap and let it chill in the refrigerator for at least 1 hour.

3. When ready to bake the cookies, pour the sesame seeds into a shallow bowl. Scoop chilled dough into generous teaspoons, roll it into balls with lightly moistened hands, drop the balls into the sesame seeds, and roll to coat. Place the dough balls on the baking sheets, about 2 inches apart, and bake for 12 to 14 minutes until the edges are browned. Using a spatula, transfer the cookies to wire racks to cool. Store in a tightly covered container.

Sweet Wine Biscuits with Sesame

MOCHA MAMAS

MAKES 2 DOZEN COOKIES

A BILLOWY MOCHA COOKIE with lots of chocolate and coffee flavor. A thin, crisp exterior while soft and light inside, with a drizzle of coffee glaze to dress her up for a night out on the town.

FOR THE COOKIES:
½ cup oil
¾ cup sugar
¼ cup almond milk
1 tablespoon ground flax seeds
2 teaspoons cornstarch
1 teaspoon pure vanilla extract
2½ teaspoons coffee extract
1½ cups all-purpose flour
½ cup unsweetened cocoa powder
½ teaspoon baking soda
¼ teaspoon salt

FOR THE DRIZZLE:
1 cup powdered sugar
2 tablespoons almond milk
½ teaspoon coffee extract
¼ teaspoon pure vanilla extract

1. Preheat oven to 350°F.
2. In a medium-size mixing bowl, vigorously stir together oil, sugar, almond milk, flax seeds, and cornstarch until thick and smooth, about 2 minutes. Mix in the extracts.
3. Sift in the remaining cookie ingredients, stirring as you add them. Once all the ingredients are added, mix until you've got a pliable dough.
4. Line two baking sheets with parchment paper. Roll the dough into walnut-size balls and pat them down just a bit onto the baking sheets. Bake for 10 to 12 minutes; they should be nice and puffy. Remove the cookies from the oven and let them cool for 5 minutes, then transfer them to wire racks to cool completely.
5. In the meantime make the drizzle. Sift the powdered sugar into a

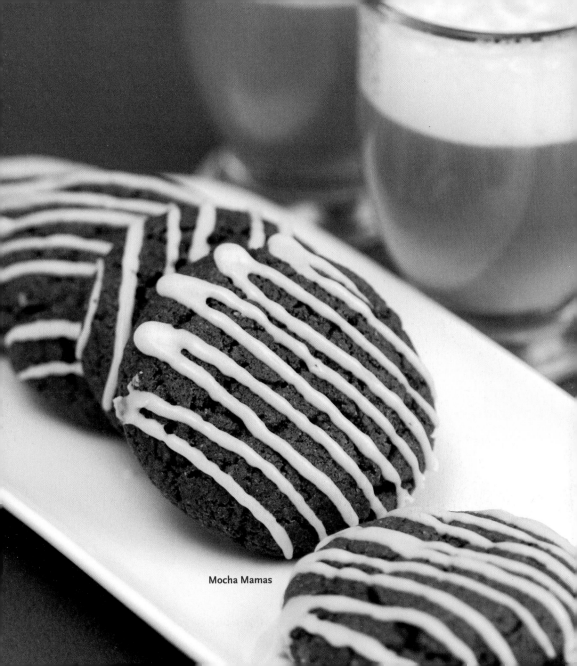

Mocha Mamas

small mixing bowl. Add the almond milk and extracts and mix vigorously with a strong fork for about 2 minutes. The drizzle should be nice and smooth and fall from the fork in ribbons. You can test to see if the consistency is right by drizzling a bit onto parchment paper. If it doesn't spread too much, you are good to go. If it seems clumpy, add a little extra almond milk by the half teaspoon. If it spreads too much, add sifted powdered sugar by the tablespoon. Transfer the drizzle into a pastry bag fit with a small round tip or into a plastic bag with a tiny hole cut out of the corner.

6. Once cookies are cooled, drizzle the icing across them in lines. Let them set in a cool dry place for at least half an hour.

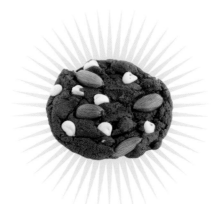

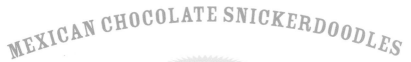

MEXICAN CHOCOLATE SNICKERDOODLES

MAKES 2 DOZEN COOKIES

TIRED OF PLAIN OLD CHOCOLATE? This is a beautiful crackle-topped chocolate cookie with a spicy cayenne kick and a sugary cinnamon coating. Sold.

FOR THE TOPPING:
- ⅓ cup sugar
- 1 teaspoon ground cinnamon

FOR THE COOKIES:
- ½ cup canola oil
- 1 cup sugar
- ¼ cup pure maple syrup
- 3 tablespoons nondairy milk
- 1 teaspoon vanilla extract
- 1 teaspoon chocolate extract (or more vanilla extract if you have no chocolate)
- 1⅔ cups all-purpose flour
- ½ cup unsweetened cocoa powder (regular, not Dutch)
- 1 teaspoon baking soda
- ¼ teaspoon salt
- ½ teaspoon cinnamon
- ½ teaspoon cayenne

1. Preheat oven to 350°F. Line two large baking sheets with parchment paper.
2. Mix the topping ingredients together on a large dinner plate. Set aside.
3. In a medium-size mixing bowl, use a fork to vigorously mix together the oil, sugar, syrup, and milk. Mix in the extracts.
4. Sift in the remaining ingredients, stirring as you add them. Once all the ingredients are added, mix until you've got a pliable dough.
5. Roll the dough into walnut-size balls. Pat the dough balls into the sugar topping to flatten into roughly 2-inch discs. Transfer the dough balls to a baking sheet, sugar

side up, at least 2 inches apart (they do spread). This should be easy as the bottom of the cookies should just stick to your fingers so you can just flip them over onto the baking sheet. Bake for 10 to 12 minutes; they should be a bit spread and crackly on top. Remove the cookies from the oven and let them cool for 5 minutes, then transfer them to wire racks to cool completely.

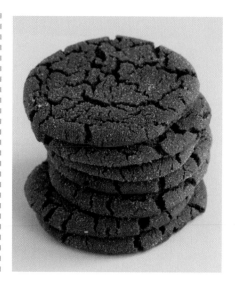

WHOLESOME COOKIES

WHILE WE LOVE A NICE SUGARY TREAT (as evidenced by every other chapter in the book), we also recognize that a little healthfulness in a snack can be scrumptious, too. Whether you're baking for a gluten-free friend or your diabetic uncle or if you just want to experiment with nutritious flours, this is the chapter for you. The supermarket shelves are filling up with alternatives to refined flours and sugars, and these recipes make great use of them; from brown rice syrup–sweetened cookies that are suitable for breakfast to agave nectar and whole wheat chocolate chip cookies to low-fat cookies that take advantage of applesauce, these are the treats for people who think that "vegan" should mean "healthy."

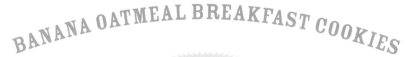

BANANA OATMEAL BREAKFAST COOKIES

MAKES 2 DOZEN LARGE COOKIES

IF YOU END UP EATING COOKIES FOR BREAKFAST like some of us do, you might as well make it these hearty lovelies. Brimming with bananas, loaded with whole grains and nuts, and gently sweetened, these cookies will give you a solid start to the day without a sugar crash come 10 a.m. Who needs scones when these big, tender cookies have all the texture, plus buckets of nutrition, and still taste great with your favorite tea or coffee? Try warming them for 10 to 15 seconds in the micro if you're not running out the door just yet.

⅔ cup well-mashed ripe banana (about two small bananas)
2 tablespoons ground flax seeds
¼ cup nondairy milk
½ cup canola oil
½ cup brown rice syrup
¼ cup agave nectar
1 teaspoon pure vanilla extract
1 cup all-purpose flour
1 cup whole wheat pastry flour
1½ teaspoons ground cinnamon
¼ teaspoon ground nutmeg
1 teaspoon baking soda
½ teaspoon salt
2 cups quick-cooking or rolled oats
1 cup pecan or walnut halves, toasted and coarsely chopped
1 cup dried cranberries

1. Preheat oven to 350°F. Line two baking sheets with parchment paper.
2. In a large mixing bowl, combine banana, flax seeds, and nondairy milk and mix until smooth. Mix in the oil, brown rice syrup, agave nectar, and vanilla. Sift in all-purpose flour, whole wheat pastry flour, cinnamon, nutmeg, baking soda, and salt and mix to form a moist batter. Fold in the oats, pecans, and dried cranberries. The dough will be moist yet thick and sticky.

3. Drop scant ¼ cups of dough about 2 inches apart onto the baking sheets. Spray the inside of the measuring cup with nonstick cooking spray to help release the dough from the cup. Use the back of a large measuring cup to press down cookies to about a 1-inch thickness.

4. Bake the cookies for 14 to 16 minutes or until edges begin to turn golden brown. Let the cookies cool on the baking sheet for 5 minutes, then transfer them to wire racks to cool completely. Store loosely covered as these cookies get rather soft if stored tightly covered. These cookies can stay fresh for up to 2 months in the freezer, just seal tightly in plastic wrap. To thaw, just let sit at room temperature for 15 minutes.

Morsels

This dough is very sticky and moist compared with typical oatmeal cookie dough, but do not fear it. The oats and flax bind everything nicely in the end.

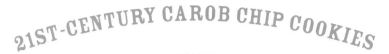
21ST-CENTURY CAROB CHIP COOKIES

MAKES 2 DOZEN LARGE COOKIES

IT'S A NEW CENTURY, so it's as good a time as ever to get (re)acquainted with the chocolate-of-the-future, otherwise known as carob. Here's our carob theory: after humankind destroys the rainforests (home to cocoa plantations world over), all we'll be left with is good old carob. That's okay, though, 'cause carob is sweet, with a toasty nuanced flavor, and deserves some love after so many years in chocolate's shadow. Enjoy "futurechocolate" with these cookies via two components: plenty of finely ground carob powder (use roasted for fullest flavor) and carob chips. Crunchy nuts and a touch of chewy currants make these fun and updated from the carob sweets of hippie days past.

⅓ cup nondairy milk
2 tablespoons ground flax seeds
½ cup canola oil
1¼ cups Sucanat or other natural dried sweetener
2 teaspoons pure vanilla extract
1½ cups whole wheat pastry flour
½ cup roasted carob powder
½ teaspoon baking soda
¼ teaspoon baking powder
½ teaspoon salt
¾ cup dairy-free carob chips
¾ cup roasted peanuts or toasted walnuts, chopped
½ cup currants or raisins

1. Preheat oven to 350°F. Line two baking sheets with parchment paper.
2. In a large mixing bowl, combine nondairy milk, flax seeds, oil, Sucanat, and vanilla. Mix until well blended and smooth. Sift in whole wheat pastry flour, carob powder, baking soda, baking powder, and salt. Stir to form a thick dough but do not overmix. Fold in carob chips, peanuts, and currants. If dough seems too sticky, chill for 30 minutes to firm up, but this step is not essential.

3. For each cookie, roll about 2 tablespoons of dough into a ball and press onto the baking sheet, placing cookies 2 inches apart, as they will spread. Bake for 8 to 10 minutes, until spread and cracked on top. Let the cookies cool on the baking sheet for 5 minutes, then transfer them to wire racks to cool completely. Store in a loosely covered container.

✳ *Morsels* ✳

Keep your eyes peeled for vegan carob chips, as some carob chips may contain dairy. Vegan carob chips can be a little bit melty after baking so we really recommend using parchment paper for these.

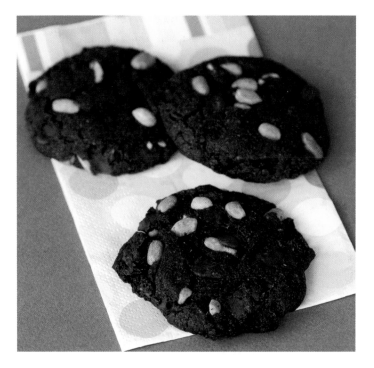

CHOCOLATE AGAVE TRAILMIXERS

MAKES 2 DOZEN COOKIES

WHEN YOU WANT CHOCOLATE and want it with a touch of innocence. These soft, chocolaty nuggets are enriched with whole wheat pastry flour, sweetened with wholesome agave nectar, and loaded with the trailmix-worthy combo of chocolate chips, peanuts or walnuts, and dried cherries (or raisins, if that's what you're into).

¼ cup nondairy milk
1 tablespoon ground flax seeds
⅔ cup canola oil
¾ cup agave nectar
2 teaspoons pure vanilla extract
½ teaspoon almond extract
1¼ cups all-purpose flour
¾ cup whole wheat pastry flour
½ cup cocoa powder
¾ teaspoon baking soda
A generous ¼ teaspoon salt
½ cup chocolate chips
½ cup whole roasted peanuts, toasted walnuts, or roasted cashews
½ cup dried cherries or raisins

1. Preheat oven to 325°F. Line two baking sheets with parchment paper.

2. In a large bowl, whisk together nondairy milk, flax seeds, oil, agave nectar, vanilla extract, and almond extract until combined, about 2 minutes. Sift in all-purpose flour, whole wheat pastry flour, cocoa powder, baking soda, and salt and mix to form a soft dough. Fold in the chocolate chips, nuts, and dried fruit.

3. For each cookie drop about 2 tablespoons of dough, 2 inches apart, onto the baking sheets. If the dough is sticking spray the spoon or dough scoop with nonstick spray. If desired, lightly flatten cookies with the back of a measuring cup sprayed with nonstick spray.

4. Bake for 12 to 14 minutes, until firm. Let the cookies cool on a baking sheet for 5 minutes, then transfer them to wire racks to cool completely. Store in a tightly covered container.

Variation

ESPRESSO-KISSED CHOCOLATE AGAVE TRAIL-MIXERS: Whisk in 1 tablespoon of instant espresso powder to the liquid ingredients before adding the dry stuff. The espresso subtly enhances and deepens the cocoa flavor.

Morsels

For easier measuring of agave nectar, measure oil first in measuring cup, then measure the agave nectar right after. The slick oiled surface of the cup will help make the agave slide out easily.

ORANGE AGAVE CHOCOLATE CHIP COOKIES

MAKES 2 DOZEN LARGE COOKIES

A WELL-BEHAVED CHOCOLATE CHIP COOKIE with some whole wheat flour goodness and a lively touch of fresh orange flavor. Agave nectar gives this cookie (and any agave-sweetened cookie) a unique, just-cakey-enough texture: pleasingly soft in the center, firm and crisp along the edges. A perfect cookie to make if you've always wanted to bake with agave but didn't know where to start.

⅔ cup agave nectar
⅔ cup canola oil
2 tablespoons nondairy milk
1 tablespoon ground flax seeds
1½ teaspoons pure vanilla extract
Grated zest of one orange (about 1 tablespoon of zest)
1½ cups all-purpose flour
1 cup whole wheat pastry flour
¾ teaspoon baking soda
A generous ¼ teaspoon salt
1 cup chocolate chips (use grain-sweetened to keep them refined-sugar-free)

1. Preheat oven to 325°F. Line two baking sheets with parchment paper.

2. In a large bowl, whisk together agave nectar, oil, nondairy milk, flax seeds, vanilla, and orange zest until smooth, about 2 minutes. Sift in the all-purpose flour, whole wheat pastry flour, baking soda, and salt and mix to form a soft dough. Fold in the chocolate chips.

3. Drop generously rounded tablespoons of dough 2 inches apart onto the baking sheets. Bake cookies for 12 to 14 minutes, until the edges are golden. Let the cookies cool on the baking sheet for 5 minutes, then transfer to wire racks to cool completely. Store in a tightly covered container.

PEANUT BUTTER AGAVE COOKIES

MAKES 2 DOZEN COOKIES

ANOTHER GREAT COOKIE that bypasses refined sugars in favor of everyone's favorite succulent-based sweetener. Agave nectar does this cookie right, giving it just enough sweetness and a firm, biscuity texture. And a little brown rice syrup adds caramel notes to boost the peanut butter flavor. These guys look great with the traditional cross-hatched peanut butter cookie shape but are equally at home with some grain-sweetened chocolate chips in the mix.

½ cup agave nectar
¼ cup brown rice syrup
⅓ cup canola oil
⅔ cup creamy or chunky salted peanut butter
2 tablespoons nondairy milk
1 tablespoon ground flax seeds
2 teaspoons pure vanilla extract
¼ teaspoon almond extract
1½ cups all-purpose flour
¾ cup whole wheat pastry flour
1 teaspoon baking soda
A generous ¼ teaspoon salt

1. Preheat oven to 325°F. Line two baking sheets with parchment paper.
2. In a large bowl, whisk together the agave nectar, brown rice syrup, oil, peanut butter, nondairy milk, flax seeds, and vanilla and almond extracts until smooth, about 3 minutes. Sift in the all-purpose flour, whole wheat pastry flour, baking soda, and salt and mix to form a soft dough.
3. Drop large, generously rounded tablespoons of dough 2 inches apart onto the baking sheets. Flatten the cookies to about 1 inch using the

back of a measuring cup. Lightly spray the back of the cup with non-stick spray if the dough starts to stick. Then use a fork to press a crosshatch pattern onto the tops of cookies, spraying with cooking spray to prevent sticking if necessary.

4. Bake the cookies for 12 to 14 minutes, until the edges are golden. Let the cookies cool on the baking sheet for 5 minutes, then transfer them to wire racks to cool completely. Store in a tightly covered container.

Variation

PEANUT BUTTER CHOCOLATE CHIP: Fold in 1 cup of grain-sweetened chocolate chips into cookie dough before baking.

Morsels

If all you have is
unsalted peanut butter,
up the salt to
½ teaspoon.

FRUITY OATY BARS

NOT TOO SWEET OR WEIGHED DOWN with junky stuff, these Fruity Oaty Bars are tightly packed with energy like a flying fist! Sturdy yet chewy, featuring no refined sugar and tons of whole grains, fruits, and seeds, these bars will keep you jazzed while ridding the universe of cannibalistic interstellar barbarian hordes. Or while biking, hiking, or other activities people apparently do in this "outside" we keep hearing about.

The mandatory elements of pepitas and dried cranberries make these bars look festive, but you can play with the flavor by adding some additional citrus zest, dried coconut, or bite-size bits of any dried fruits. Try adding apricots for tangy, fresh flavor or dried pineapple for a sweet and mellow treat that lets the other ingredients' flavors shine through.

3 cups old-fashioned rolled oats
1½ cups spelt flour
½ cup wheat germ
1 teaspoon cinnamon
½ teaspoon baking soda
½ teaspoon salt
½ cup orange juice
3 tablespoons ground flax seeds
1 teaspoon pure vanilla extract
½ cup canola oil
⅔ cup brown rice syrup
¼ cup barley malt syrup
½ cup sesame seeds
½ cup pepitas or sunflower seeds
½ cup dried cranberries

1 cup dried chopped fruit, such as pineapple, apricots, apples, golden raisins, dates, papaya, or a mix

1. Preheat oven to 350°F. Line a 9 x 13-inch baking pan that has at least a 2-inch rim with parchment paper.
2. In a large bowl, combine rolled oats, spelt flour, wheat germ, cinnamon, baking soda, and salt. In a separate bowl or large measuring cup, whisk together orange juice

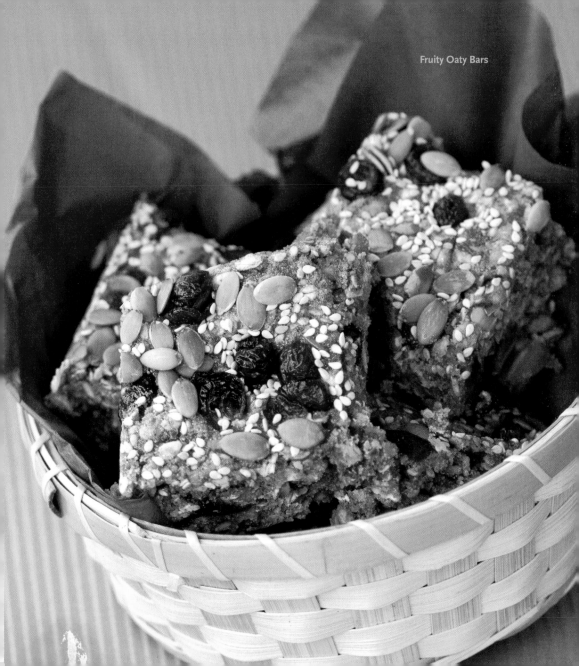

and flax seeds, then mix in the vanilla, oil, brown rice syrup, and barley malt syrup until smooth.

3. Form a well in the center of the dry ingredients and pour in the orange juice mixture. Using a rubber spatula, stir to moisten the ingredients, then fold in sesame seeds, pepitas, cranberries, and dried fruit. The dough will be very sticky and thick; you may want to fold in these last ingredients using your hands.

4. Use lightly moistened hands to firmly and evenly press the dough into the prepared baking pan. Take care that the dough in the center of the pan is not too thick; press the dough slightly toward the edges of the pan. Bake for 26 to 28 minutes until the top is golden brown and firm.

5. Remove the pan from the oven and place it on a wire rack to cool. Let it cool for at least 45 minutes, then use a thin, very sharp serrated knife to carefully cut 16 bars. Store the bars in a tightly covered container, or wrap them individually tightly in foil and freeze.

Variations

FRUITY OATY COCONUTTY BARS: Add 1 cup unsweetened, grated coconut along with oats.

ORANGE-KISSED FRUITY OATY BARS: For bigger orange flavor, add the finely grated zest of one large orange when adding the wet ingredients.

APPLESAUCE SOFTIES

MAKES 2 DOZEN COOKIES

IF "WHOLESOME" IS WHY YOU FLIPPED to this chapter, then you've come to the right page. While a casual cookie eater may not detect a strong apple taste here, the pleasant combination of whole grains and fruit will keep the health enthusiast in your life happy. Or at least away from your stash of chocolate chip cookies.

Applesauce is a favorite ingredient in lots of healthy baked goods. We enjoy it as much as the next gal but crave a cookie that's not too moist or crumbly, as applesaucy cookies often are. This recipe borrows the reducing technique from the SELL YOUR SOUL PUMPKIN COOKIES (page 51) for tender yet toothsome cookies. Try experimenting with applesauce cooked down to varying degrees for different cookie consistencies.

1⅓ cups natural unsweetened applesauce
⅓ cup canola oil
¾ cup Sucanat or other granulated natural sweetener
1 teaspoon pure vanilla extract
A large pinch of finely grated lemon rind
1 cup whole wheat pastry flour
¾ cup all-purpose flour
1 tablespoon cornstarch
1 teaspoon ground cinnamon
¼ teaspoon ground nutmeg
¼ teaspoon ground cloves
½ teaspoon baking soda
¼ teaspoon salt

Optional Cinnamon Sugar topping:
3 tablespoons Sucanat or other granulated natural sweetener mixed with ½ teaspoon ground cinnamon

1. To reduce the applesauce, cook it in a saucepan over medium heat for about 25 minutes, stirring often. Keep the heat low enough that it doesn't rapidly boil, but instead appears to be steaming and occasionally bubbling. After about 20 minutes spoon the applesauce into

a measuring cup to measure how much it has reduced. It should measure about ⅔ cup by now. If not, return it to the pot to continue cooking until it has reduced to ⅔ cup or slightly less. When done, remove the saucepan from the heat and let the applesauce cool completely before proceeding.

2. Preheat oven to 350°F. Line two baking sheets with parchment paper.

3. In a large mixing bowl, stir together the oil, Sucanat, vanilla, and lemon rind. Mix in the cooled applesauce, then sift in the whole wheat pastry flour, all-purpose flour, cinnamon, nutmeg, cloves, baking soda, and salt. Mix to form a soft dough.

4. For each cookie, scoop 1 rounded tablespoon of dough onto a baking sheet, keeping the cookies about 2 inches apart. Sprinkle with a little Cinnamon Sugar if using and flatten the tops with the back of a measuring cup. Bake the cookies for 8 to 10 minutes or until puffed and just starting to brown on the edges. Remove the cookies from the oven and let them cool on the baking sheet for 5 minutes before transferring them to wire racks to cool completely.

Variations

APPLE WALNUT SOFTIES: Fold ½ cup finely chopped walnuts into the dough.

APPLE RAISIN SOFTIES: Prior to making dough, soak 1 cup raisins in ½ cup apple juice or apple cider for 30 minutes or until plump. Drain raisins well of excess apple juice, then fold them into the dough.

WHOLE WHEAT CHOCOLATE CHIP COOKIES

MAKES 2 DOZEN COOKIES

WHEN YOU WANT TO HAVE YOUR CHOCOLATE CHIP COOKIE and eat it, too, this is a great go-to cookie. It's made with white whole wheat flour for that "but-I-swear-to-god-it's-healthy" feeling. White whole wheat gives great texture—a little cakier than your usual chocolate chipper, yet it's still got a nice bite to it.

⅓ cup sugar
⅓ cup brown sugar
½ cup canola oil
½ cup almond milk (or your nondairy milk of choice)
2 tablespoons tapioca flour (you can sub arrowroot powder or cornstarch)
2 teaspoons pure vanilla extract
2 cups white whole wheat flour
½ teaspoon baking soda
½ teaspoon salt
1 cup semisweet chocolate chips

1. Preheat oven to 350°F.
2. In a mixing bowl, mix together the sugars and oil for about a minute. You want to get the sugars a bit broken down. Add the almond milk and tapioca flour and beat vigorously until there are no clumps of tapioca left. Mix in the vanilla.
3. Add half the flour, the baking soda, and salt and mix well. Mix in the remaining flour. Fold in the chocolate chips.
4. Drop dough by rounded tablespoon onto baking sheets lined with parchment paper, or lightly greased. Space the cookies about 2 inches apart and flatten them down a bit with your fingers.

5. Bake 10 minutes for soft, chewy cookies, 12 minutes for crispier ones. When they're done baking, let the cookies rest on the sheets for about 5 minutes before transferring them to wire racks to finish cooling.

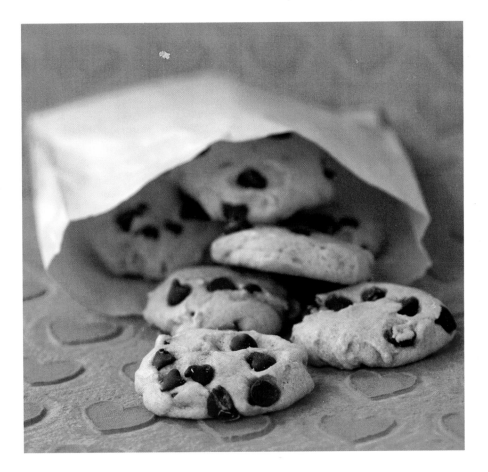

WHOLESOME COOKIES

APRICOT ALMOND QUINOA CHEWS

MAKES 2 DOZEN COOKIES

TART-SWEET DRIED APRICOTS, crunchy almonds, and quinoa in two forms make beautiful music together in these nutritious, chewy-crisp gems that are also gluten-free. Quinoa flour is an excellent wheat flour alternative if gluten-free baking is what you seek, and the addition of quick-cooking quinoa flakes gives boatloads of pleasantly grainy texture and flavor.

½ cup nondairy milk
2 tablespoons ground flax seeds
⅓ cup canola oil
⅔ cup sugar
1 teaspoon pure vanilla extract
½ cup quinoa flour
½ cup brown rice flour
2 tablespoons tapioca flour or arrowroot powder
½ teaspoon ground cinnamon
½ teaspoon ground cardamom
½ teaspoon baking soda
¼ teaspoon salt
1 cup quick-cooking quinoa flakes
½ cup finely chopped dried apricots
¼ cup sliced almonds
Additional sliced almonds for decorating cookies

1. Preheat oven to 350°F. Line two baking sheets with parchment paper.

2. In a large mixing bowl, whisk together the nondairy milk and flax seeds and let sit for 1 minute. Then stir in the sugar and vanilla until smooth. Sift in the quinoa flour, brown rice flour, tapioca flour, cinnamon, cardamom, baking soda, and salt. Mix to form a thick batter, then fold in the quinoa flakes, apricots, and almonds.

3. For each cookie scoop 1 rounded tablespoon of dough onto the baking sheet, keeping the cookies about 2 inches apart. Sprinkle the

cookie tops with a few sliced almonds and flatten the tops with the back of a measuring cup. Bake for 10 to 12 minutes or until puffed and just starting to brown on the edges. Remove the cookies from the oven and let them cool on the cookie sheet for 5 minutes. Transfer them to wire racks to cool completely and store in a tightly covered container. These cookies are best eaten the day they are made.

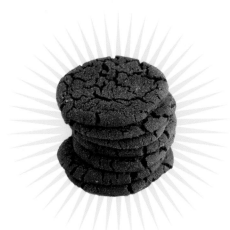

BAR COOKIES

AS IF COOKIES WEREN'T ALREADY EASY ENOUGH! Whoever came up with the idea of confining delicious cookies to a fun and easy bar shape must have been a very lazy genius. Vegan cookie lovers can honor these pioneers of cookie technology every day with this delightful assortment of bars. Start it up with two kinds of brownies to choose from, three blondies (sweet potato even!), and a caramel pecan bar to die for. Not to mention the joyous cries of "I can't believe it's vegan!" you'll hear after you serve MAGICAL COCONUT COOKIE BARS (page 121) or LEMON BARS (page 141). You'll just have to reply, "Yes you can, because vegan bars rock. Sheesh." Since there's only one "batch" to bake with bar cookies, you get big results with less effort.

CARAMEL PECAN BARS

DEEP, DARK, BROWN RICE CARAMEL, lots of crunchy pecans, and a buttery crust. What else is there left to talk about? A huge hit with our testers, these bars were reported to have the power to win friends and influence people ... so put down the self-help book and get baking!

These bars are a little stickier than most bar cookies so you may want to store them in their baking pan until it's time to serve. For an oh-so-hip 'n' current variation, sprinkle the top ever so lightly with your favorite gourmet coarse-grained salt for (you guessed it) Salted Caramel Pecan Bars.

FOR THE CRUST:
- 2 cups all-purpose flour
- ⅓ cup dark brown sugar
- ¼ teaspoon ground cinnamon
- ¼ teaspoon baking powder
- A big pinch of salt
- ¾ cup nonhydrogenated margarine, slightly softened

FOR THE PECAN TOPPING:
- 3 tablespoons cornstarch
- ⅓ cup nondairy milk
- 1½ cups dark brown sugar
- ⅔ cup brown rice syrup
- 2 tablespoons melted nonhydrogenated margarine
- 2 teaspoons pure vanilla extract
- ¼ teaspoon salt
- 2 cups coarsely chopped pecans

1. Preheat oven to 350°F. Line a 9 x 13 x 2-inch baking pan with aluminum foil, making sure the foil completely covers the sides of the pan, with about 2 inches folded outside over the edges. Spray the bottom and sides of the pan generously with nonstick cooking spray.

PREPARE THE CRUST:

1. In a mixing bowl, combine the flour, brown sugar, cinnamon, baking

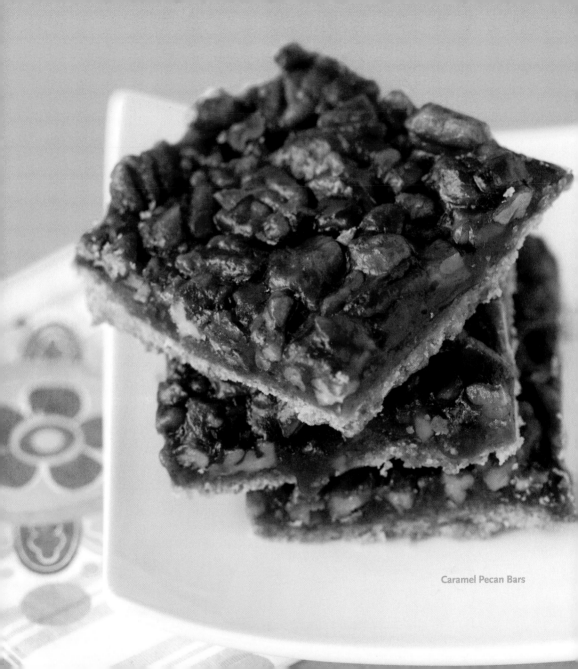

Caramel Pecan Bars

powder, and salt. Use a pastry cutter or two knives held together to cut in the margarine until mixture resembles fine crumbs. Pour crumbs into the prepared baking pan and press down evenly and very firmly, making sure to press the mixture all the way to the edges of the pan. Bake the crust for 8 to 10 minutes until firm and very lightly browned. Remove the pan from the oven and set it aside.

PREPARE THE TOPPING:

1. In a large bowl, whisk together the cornstarch and nondairy milk until foamy. Stir in the dark brown sugar, brown rice syrup, melted margarine, vanilla, and salt until smooth. Fold in the pecans and pour the mixture onto the crust, using a spatula to spread the topping evenly.

2. Return the pan to the oven and bake for 28 to 30 minutes, or until the filling is rapidly bubbling. Place the pan on a wire rack to cool for 20 minutes, then move it to the refrigerator to finish cooling and setting. Chill for at least 2 hours or, even better, overnight.

3. To slice completely cooled bars, grab ahold of the foil and carefully lift the whole thing out of the pan and onto a heavy cutting board. Peel away the foil and cut bars with a heavy, sharp knife.

Variation

SALTED CARAMEL PECAN BARS: Right after the bars are out of the oven and the topping is still hot, sprinkle the surface very sparingly with your favorite coarse-grained gourmet salt. Cool and slice as directed.

BLUEBERRY SPICE CRUMB BARS

MAKES 12 BARS

THESE BARS ARE THE PERFECT SNACK FOR ... just about anytime! A shortbread crust, a layer of sweet blueberries, all covered in a crumb topping and spiked with warm spices. Spelt flour makes for a beautifully homey and rustic crumb, plus provides a nice home-y taste.

These cookies are also deceptively easy to make. The crust and topping are the same batter, just applied in different ways, and the blueberry filling bakes right in between—no need to mess up a million bowls.

FOR THE CRUST AND TOPPING:

3 cups spelt flour
1 cup sugar
1 teaspoon baking powder
2 teaspoons ground cinnamon
2 teaspoons ground ginger
½ teaspoon ground allspice
¼ teaspoon salt
1 cup nonhydrogenated vegetable
   shortening, at room temperature
3 to 4 tablespoons nondairy milk

FOR THE BLUEBERRY FILLING:

16 ounces (about 4 cups) fresh or
   frozen blueberries
½ cup sugar
4 teaspoons cornstarch

2 tablespoons cold water
1 teaspoon pure vanilla extract

1. Preheat oven to 350°F. Lightly grease a 9 x 13-inch baking pan.
2. In a medium-size mixing bowl, stir together the flour, sugar, baking powder, spices, and salt. Add the shortening by the spoonful, cutting it into the flour with a pastry cutter or two knives held together. Once the dough becomes crumbly, add the nondairy milk by the tablespoon. Use your fingers to stir the milk in after each addition until pea-size crumbs form.

3. In a separate bowl, stir together the blueberries, sugar, cornstarch, water, and vanilla.

4. Scoop 3 cups of the dough into the prepared baking pan. Firmly press it in to form the base of the bars. Spread the blueberry mixture over the base and then sprinkle the rest of the crumbly dough over the blueberries.

5. Bake for about 45 minutes. When ready, the blueberries should be nice and bubbly. Cool completely before cutting into bars and eating.

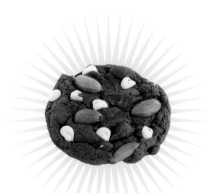

WHOLE WHEAT FIG BARS

MAKES 12 BARS

SOFT, FLAVORFUL, FIG-FILLED SQUARES get extra-healthy props with a tender whole wheat crust sweetened with goody-two-shoes Sucanat (or any dry natural sweetener you like). Moisture-rich, fruity cookies like these really do taste better the next day. So bake these the night before, wrap them up tight and go to bed looking forward to a figgy new day.

FOR THE FIG FILLING:
- 1 pound dried figs, preferably Black Mission, hard stems removed and diced into small pieces
- ⅔ cup water
- ¼ cup agave nectar or maple syrup
- 2 teaspoons finely grated citrus zest (try lemon, orange, lime or a combination)

FOR THE DOUGH:
- 2 tablespoons ground flax seeds
- ¼ cup nondairy milk
- ½ cup canola oil
- ¾ cup Sucanat or other natural dry sweetener
- 1½ teaspoons pure vanilla extract
- 1¾ cups whole wheat pastry flour
- ½ teaspoon baking powder
- ½ teaspoon baking soda
- ½ teaspoon salt

1. Line an 8 x 8-inch square metal brownie pan with enough aluminum foil so that it folds over the sides of the pan by about an inch. Spray the bottom of the covered pan with a little nonstick cooking spray. Preheat oven to 350°F.

2. In a large saucepan, combine figs, water, agave nectar, and citrus zest. Bring to boil over medium heat, reduce to a simmer, and stir occasionally. When the figs begin to soften in about 8 to 10 minutes, continue to cook but mash the figs with a firm spatula or a fork to create a chunky, moist paste. If mixture starts to look overly dry, add 2 tablespoons of water and stir,

Whole Wheat Fig Bars

dribbling additional water into the mixture if necessary. Remove the filling from the heat and set aside. If the mixture still seems too chunky, puree it in a food processor until a smooth texture is reached.

3. In a large mixing bowl, combine flax seeds, nondairy milk, oil, Sucanat, and vanilla until smooth, mixing for about 1½ minutes. Sift in whole wheat pastry flour, baking powder, baking soda, and salt. Stir to form a soft dough and divide into two equal parts. Shape each section of dough into a square shape; next you'll be rolling the square out.

4. Place one square of dough between two large sheets of waxed paper. With a rolling pin roll the dough into a larger square about the same size as the 8 x 8-inch pan (slightly larger is fine). Occasionally rotate the dough while rolling to help maintain an even thickness.

5. When finished rolling peel off the top layer of waxed paper and flip the dough directly into the prepared baking pan. Remove the top

layer of waxed paper and press the dough firmly into the pan. Spread all the fig filling over the dough, making sure to evenly cover all the way to the edges. Prepare the top crust with the remaining dough using the same method as the bottom crust, flipping it on top of the filling and pressing the dough evenly and all the way to the edges.

6. Bake for 20 to 22 minutes until crust is golden and puffed. Remove the pan from the oven and place it on a wire rack to cool. When completely cool, grabbing the edges of the foil, lift everything out of the pan and flip it over onto a cutting board. Peel off the foil and slice into 12 bars. Store in a tightly covered container.

☀ *Morsels* ☀

Not all dried figs are created equal, and some may require adding more water than mentioned in the recipe. You'll want to cook them with just enough liquid to create a moist, thick, but not too stiff filling.

(FOR THE LOVE OF) FRUITCAKE BARS

MAKES 2 DOZEN SNACK CAKE BARS

TRUE FRUITCAKE LOVERS DON'T MIND all the trash-talking this morsel gets during the holidays. More for us, never mind the haters. But sometimes even a diehard fan doesn't want to commit to baking an entire loaf, so these dainties provide all the fruity, nutty, and spicy goodness (with a touch of rum) in two- or three-bite portions. They're a little more cake-like than cookie-like and make a rich, festive bar when you want something beyond brownies. Just like real fruitcake, the flavor of these bars improves when given time to develop, so try baking these the day before serving and store them in a tightly covered container. They freeze well, too; just hold off on the glaze topping until after they've thawed.

1 cup golden raisins
1 cup mixed candied fruit or mixed
   chopped glacé fruit, packed
½ cup candied ginger, finely chopped
¼ cup dark or spiced rum
⅓ cup canola oil
¾ cup brown sugar, firmly packed
¼ cup freshly squeezed orange juice
⅓ cup nondairy milk
1 tablespoon grated orange rind
1⅔ cups all-purpose flour
1 tablespoon cocoa powder (natural or
   Dutch)
1 teaspoon baking powder
½ teaspoon baking soda
½ teaspoon salt

1½ teaspoons ground cinnamon
½ teaspoon ground nutmeg
½ teaspoon ground allspice
¼ teaspoon ground cloves
1 cup pecans or walnuts, toasted and
   chopped

FOR THE GLAZE:
⅔ cup powdered sugar, sifted
1 tablespoon rum
2 to 3 teaspoons orange juice

1. In a small bowl, combine the raisins, fruit, ginger, and rum. Let stand for at least 30 minutes or for up to 2 hours, stirring occasionally to allow the fruit to absorb more rum.

2. Preheat oven to 350°F. Line a 9 x 13 x 2-inch baking pan with parchment paper.

3. In a large bowl, mix together the oil, brown sugar, orange juice, nondairy milk, and orange rind until smooth. Sift in the flour, cocoa powder, baking powder, baking soda, salt, cinnamon, nutmeg, allspice, and cloves. Stir until the dry ingredients are moistened, then fold in the rum-marinated fruits and the pecans. Take care not to overmix.

4. Spread the dough into the prepared baking pan and bake for 28 to 30 minutes, until a toothpick inserted into the center of the cake comes out clean. Remove the pan from the oven and place it on a wire rack to cool, about an hour.

5. To make the glaze: In a medium-size bowl, use either an electric mixer or a fork to combine powdered sugar with rum. Then stir in the orange juice, one teaspoon at a time, until you have a thin, smooth glaze.

6. Use a fork to drizzle the glaze on the completely cooled cake and allow the glaze to set before slicing, at least 45 minutes. Use a very sharp knife to slice the cake into 24 bars and lift the bars out of the pan with a spatula. Store in a tightly covered container.

7. To freeze: Wrap the unsliced, unglazed cake tightly with plastic wrap, then with foil, and freeze. To serve, thaw the cake for about half an hour, then glaze and slice.

✴ Morsels ✴

◆ Regular old "mixed candied fruit," the kind that appears in groceries during the winter holidays, is ideal in this recipe. But if you want something a little more upscale and without the fake green and red bits, try using glacé fruits—candied pears, prunes, and apricots are all over the place this time of year. Just be sure to chop them small, under ¼ inch or so.

◆ Try using any brandy instead of rum!

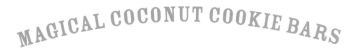

MAGICAL COCONUT COOKIE BARS

MAKES 24 VERY RICH LITTLE BARS

AS THE SONG FROM *XANADU* (THE MOVIE) GOES, "you have to believe we are magic," and nothing will stand in your way once you taste this unapologetically vegan version that dreams are made of. Here are the nutty, chocolaty, ultra-sweet, and buttery-tasting graham-cracker coconut bars you loved so much as a kid. If your childhood was lacking in magical moments like these bars, then these are tastier than therapy for sure. The vegan secret weapon of choice here is cooked-down coconut milk, which brings in even bigger coconut flavor than ever imagined. Should you get your hands on some ever-elusive vegan butterscotch chips, they make a sublime addition.

These bars require a good overnight chilling to really firm them up before slicing, so plan accordingly.

One 14-ounce can (regular or light) coconut milk (about 1¾ cups)
⅔ cup dark brown sugar
2 cups graham cracker crumbs
½ cup melted nonhydrogenated margarine
2 tablespoons sugar
1½ cups chocolate chips or chocolate chunks
2 cups flaked, sweetened coconut
1 cup walnuts or pecans, chopped

1. In a large saucepan, whisk together the coconut milk and brown sugar over medium-high heat. Bring to a boil, reduce heat to low, and simmer for 10 minutes, stirring occasionally. The mixture may form a thin skin on the surface; just stir it back into the liquid. Remove the mixture from the heat and let it cool while preparing the crust.

2. Preheat oven to 350°F. Line a 13 x 9 x 2-inch baking pan with parchment paper. In a large bowl, combine graham cracker crumbs, margarine, and sugar; mix well to

Magical Coconut Cookie Bars

moisten the crumbs completely. Firmly press the mixture into the prepared pan, pressing evenly from the center to the sides of the pan.

3. Pour the warm coconut milk mixture evenly over crumb base. Top with an even layer of chocolate chips, coconut, and nuts, in that order. Firmly pat everything down until the coconut milk mixture soaks upward into the toppings.

4. Bake for 28 to 30 minutes or until coconut is deeply golden and the filling is bubbling. Remove the pan from the oven and let it cool on a wire rack for 15 minutes. Transfer the pan to the refrigerator to completely cool and firm up the bars for at least 4 hours, or even better, overnight or until very firm. Run a sharp, heavy knife along the edges of the pan and slide the cake on its parchment paper out of the pan and onto a cutting board. Then, slice it into 24 squares. Store in a covered container in the refrigerator. These bars also freeze well, tightly wrapped and allowed to thaw for 20 minutes before serving.

❋ Morsels ❋

+ You'll want to use only sweetened, fluffy, white flaked coconut for these. Save the natural shredded stuff for a healthy curry.
+ Press the graham cracker crumb crust like crazy into the pan; the more you pat it down the firmer the resulting crust will be.

CALL ME BLONDIES

WE'RE NOT MUSIC HISTORIANS, but could it be that Deborah Harry named her band after this chewy, gooey bar? This is a nice and easy basic blondie, quick to throw together and packed with chocolate chips. The secret to the texture is not to overbake; once the edges are lightly browned these babies are done.

3 ounces firm silken tofu, like Mori-Nu
 (¼ of the package)
¼ cup nondairy milk
⅓ cup canola oil
½ cup brown sugar
½ cup sugar
1 teaspoon pure vanilla extract
1½ cups all-purpose flour
½ teaspoon baking soda
¼ teaspoon baking powder
½ teaspoon salt
¾ cup chocolate chips

1. Preheat oven to 325°F. Line an 8 x 8-inch brownie pan with parchment paper; it should cover the bottom as well as curve up and cover the sides.

2. Puree the tofu, nondairy milk, and oil in a blender or a food processor until smooth and fluffy. Use a spatula to scrape down the sides to make sure you get everything.

3. Transfer the tofu mixture to a mixing bowl. Use a fork to vigorously mix in the sugars. Add the vanilla.

4. Sift in the flour, baking soda, baking powder, and salt. Use a spatula to fold and mix the batter until smooth. Fold in the chocolate chips. Transfer the batter to the pan and smooth out the top. It's okay if the batter doesn't sink all the way into the sides and edges of pan, as it will spread a bit during baking. Bake for 27 to 30 minutes; the sides

of the blondies should be just slightly browned. Remove the pan from the oven and let the blondies cool for at least 30 minutes before slicing and serving.

Variations

These really are a great base for almost any combo you can imagine.

TRIPLE BLONDE BLONDIES: Add ¾ cups white chocolate chips and ¾ cup macadamia nuts.

WALNUT CHOCOLATE CHIP BLONDIES: Add ¾ cups walnuts in addition to the chocolate chips.

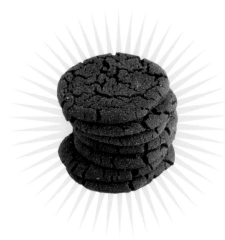

SPICED SWEET POTATO BLONDIES

BLONDIE PURISTS MAY FROWN AT THE IDEA. But sweet potato fans will welcome with open arms the lush, dense moistness that sweet potatoes bring to this old favorite. Add some chocolate chips if you must, but try the recipe without 'em sometime for really gorgeous sweet potato flavor. These plump squares are a tad more cakelike and certainly moister than your average blondie, but it also helps them remain fresher-tasting for longer.

¾ cup cooked, well-mashed, orange-colored sweet potato (less than a 1 pound of raw potato)
½ cup canola oil
⅔ cup sugar
½ cup dark brown sugar
¼ cup nondairy milk
2 teaspoons vanilla
1¼ cups unbleached flour
¼ teaspoon baking powder
¼ teaspoon salt
1 teaspoon ground cinnamon
½ teaspoon ground ginger
¼ teaspoon ground allspice
½ cup toasted chopped pecans or walnuts
½ cup chocolate chips (optional)

1. Line an 8 x 8-inch square metal brownie pan with enough aluminum foil so that it folds over the sides of the pan by about an inch. Spray the bottom of the covered pan with a little nonstick cooking spray. Preheat oven to 350°F.

2. In a large bowl, mix together the sweet potato, oil, sugar, brown sugar, nondairy milk, and vanilla until smooth. A few tiny chunks of sweet potato are okay.

3. Sift in the flour, baking powder, salt, cinnamon, ginger, and allspice. Mix just enough to moisten, then fold in the nuts and chocolate chips, if using. Do not overmix.

4. Pour mixture into the prepared pan and smooth the top with a rubber spatula. Bake for 28 to 32 minutes, checking the bars at 28 minutes by poking a toothpick into the center of the cake. Bars are done if a toothpick comes out mostly clean; a few moist crumbles here and there are okay. Take care not to overbake. Allow the blondies to cool at least 30 minutes for the texture and flavor to fully develop, then slice into 12 bars. Store in a covered container.

Morsels

A regular old fork is probably the best sweet potato mashing device ever made. Just mash away until it's as creamy as you can get it.

Peanut Butter Blondies

PEANUT BUTTER BLONDIES

MAKES 12 BLONDIES

DO YOU LIKE YOUR DESSERTS PEANUT-BUTTERY? We mean really *really* peanut-buttery? This is a beautifully rich—and dare we say *fudgy*—peanut butter blondie that is sure to please anyone with peanuts for taste buds. You'll definitely need a cup of almond milk to wash these babies down.

¾ cup peanut butter (see note)
⅓ cup oil
1 cup brown sugar
¼ cup nondairy milk
2 teaspoons pure vanilla extract
1 cup all-purpose flour
½ teaspoon salt
½ teaspoon baking powder
⅓ cup peanuts

1. Preheat oven to 350°F. Lightly grease a metal 8 x 8-inch baking dish.
2. In a mixing bowl, use a fork to vigorously mix together peanut butter, oil, and sugar. Stir in the nondairy milk and vanilla. Stir in the flour, salt, and baking powder. Once you get the flour somewhat mixed in, it's easier to just use your hands to knead the dough until soft. It will be very very thick and won't spread on its own. Transfer dough to the baking pan and press it into place. Sprinkle on the peanuts and lightly press them into the top.
3. Bake for 22 to 25 minutes; the blondie edges should be just barely darkened. The top will appear soft, and that's okay. Remove the blondies from the oven and cool completely before slicing.

❋ Morsels ❋

We used a salted, no-stir creamy peanut butter here, but a very well stirred natural peanut butter in which the oil has been incorporated should work as well. If you prefer chunky PB, that's cool, too.

ESPRESSO FUDGE BROWNIES

MAKES 12 BROWNIES

THIS IS A DENSE, TOTALLY-NOT-CAKEY, ULTRA-FUDGY BROWNIE that's built for sin. Don't underestimate its slim profile; it packs an espresso-flavored punch. Perfect for topping with 'nilla nondairy ice cream and chocolate sauce or for just enjoying on its own. Who would guess that such a naughty brownie would also be nice enough to call for just one mixing bowl (well, we're not counting a little measuring cup action)?

For best results, use the highest-quality semisweet baking chocolate (in bar form) you can buy, rather than chocolate chips. Speaking of chocolate chips, lots of our testers loved to throw a handful into the batter, but we think they're simply perfect without. You decide.

As with all fudgy brownies, slightly under-baking is essential. Test these brownies for doneness at the minimum suggested baking time initially. If the brownies seem a little dry even after that, the next time around try under-baking them by a minute or two.

3 ounces semisweet baking chocolate, chopped
5 tablespoons nonhydrogenated margarine
⅔ cup sugar
⅓ cup nondairy milk
1 tablespoon cornstarch
2½ to 3 teaspoons espresso powder
1 teaspoon vanilla
¾ cup plus 2 tablespoons all-purpose flour
½ teaspoon baking powder
3 tablespoons Dutch cocoa powder
A pinch of salt

1. Line an 8 x 8-inch square metal brownie pan with enough aluminum foil so that it folds over the sides of the pan by about an inch. Spray the bottom of the covered pan with a little nonstick cooking spray. Preheat oven to 350°F.

2. Place the chocolate and margarine in a large glass mixing bowl. Microwave at 50 percent power for 1½ to 2 minutes until the chocolate is soft enough to melt into the melted margarine when stirred with a rubber spatula. Stir until smooth, add the sugar, and stir again to combine.

3. In a liquid measuring cup, vigorously whisk together the nondairy milk, cornstarch, espresso powder, and vanilla until foamy. Stir this into the chocolate mixture, using the rubber spatula, until completely combined. Sift in the flour, baking powder, cocoa powder, and salt and fold into the chocolate mixture until moistened. A few small lumps are okay; do not overmix. Scrape the batter—getting as much as possible—into the prepared pan and smooth it out evenly to the edges of the pan.

4. Bake for 22 to 24 minutes or until a toothpick inserted into the center of the brownies comes out mostly clean with a few moist crumbs (but no gooey batter). Place the pan on a wire rack to cool for at least 30 minutes, if possible allowing the brownies to cool completely before serving. Slice into 12 brownies. Store in a tightly covered container.

Variations

MIDNIGHT BROWNIES: For the cocoa powder use 1 tablespoon Dutch cocoa powder plus 2 tablespoons black cocoa powder.

IN THE MINT CHOCOLATE BROWNIES: Omit espresso powder and add 1½ teaspoons peppermint extract. Especially nice when made with black cocoa powder, à la Midnight Brownies.

❋ Morsels ❋

✦ No microwave? Melt the chocolate and margarine together on your stovetop in a double boiler (see page 24 for more on melting chocolate). Proceed as directed.

✦ The easiest way to cut fudgy brownies is to use a thin plastic knife, carefully running it from end to end in the pan.

✦ If your brownies have cooled and you want to serve them warm, just microwave them at medium high power for 10 to 12 seconds.

DELUXE COCOA BROWNIES

MAKES 12 BROWNIES

BROWNIE PURISTS WILL DELIGHT in these super moist, melt-in-your-mouth, rich cocoa brownies. These are somewhere between fudgy and cakey, reminiscent of a brownie box mix. It *is* important to sift the dry ingredients in with a sifter. Clumpy cocoa or cornstarch can ruin your precious brownie, so sift!

3 ounces firm silken tofu, like Mori-Nu
(¼ of the package)
¼ cup nondairy milk
½ cup canola oil
1 cup sugar
2 teaspoons vanilla
1 cup flour
½ cup unsweetened cocoa powder
1 tablespoon cornstarch
½ teaspoon baking powder
½ teaspoon salt

1. Preheat oven to 325°F. Line an 8 x 8-inch brownie pan with parchment paper; it should cover the bottom as well as curve up and cover the sides.

2. Puree the tofu, nondairy milk, and oil in a blender or food processor until smooth and fluffy. Use a spatula to scrape down the sides to make sure you get everything.

3. Transfer the tofu mixture to a mixing bowl. Use a fork to vigorously mix in the sugar. Add vanilla.

4. Sift in the flour, cocoa powder, cornstarch, baking powder, and salt. Use a spatula to fold and mix batter until smooth. Transfer the batter to the pan and smooth out the top. It's okay if the batter doesn't sink all the way into the sides and edges of pan, as it will spread during baking. Bake brown-

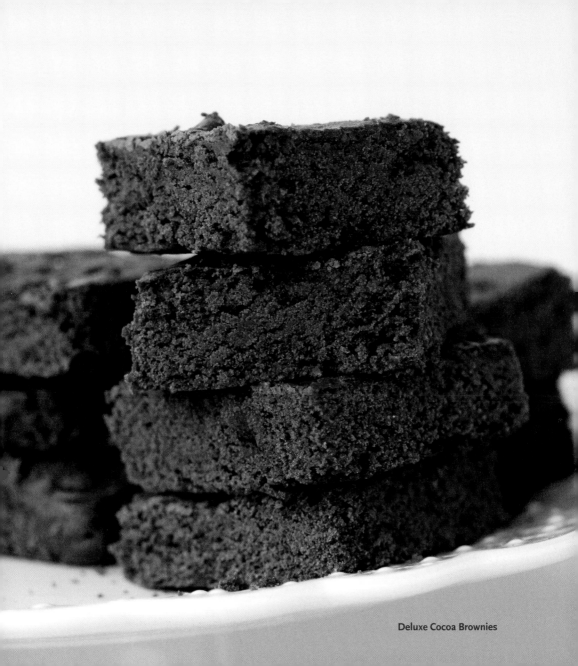

Deluxe Cocoa Brownies

ies for 30 to 32 minutes, remove the pan from the oven, and let the brownies cool for at least 15 minutes before slicing and serving.

Variations

I WANT WALNUT BROWNIES: Fold 1 cup chopped walnuts into the batter.

CHOCOLATE CHIP DELUXE BROWNIES: Fold ¾ cup chocolate chips into the batter.

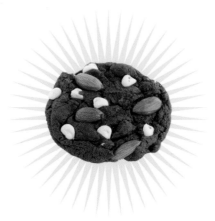

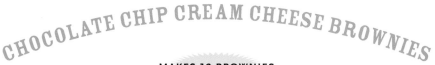

CHOCOLATE CHIP CREAM CHEESE BROWNIES

MAKES 12 BROWNIES

DELUXE COCOA BROWNIES **(PAGE 132) TRANSFORM INTO UBER-FUDGY WONDERS** when topped with a luscious, speedy-to-make cheesecakey topping. A dousing of chocolate chips makes them even more irresistible, if that's even possible. Like real cheesecake, these require a long rest in the fridge to firm up, so make these the night before brownies are required.

Prepare DELUXE COCOA BROWNIES (page 132) according to recipe directions, pouring the batter into the prepared pan and preheating the oven. Just before baking the brownies, top them with the following:

FOR THE TOPPING:

- 8 ounces plain vegan cream cheese, softened
- ½ cup sugar
- 2 tablespoons arrowroot powder
- 1 tablespoon all-purpose flour
- 1½ teaspoons vanilla
- ⅔ cup chocolate chips; use mini chips if available

1. In a large mixing bowl, using electric beaters, cream together the cream cheese and sugar until smooth. Add the arrowroot powder, flour, and vanilla and beat once more until smooth. Using a rubber spatula, scrape the entire mixture over the uncooked brownie batter, smoothing the topping evenly. Sprinkle with chocolate chips and gently stir the topping once more to distribute the chips into the topping.

2. Bake at 325°F for 35 minutes. Remove the pan from the oven and place it on a wire rack to cool. When it's cool enough to touch, place the pan in the refrigerator to chill the brownies overnight or until firm. The easiest way to slice cooled fudgy brownies is to use a

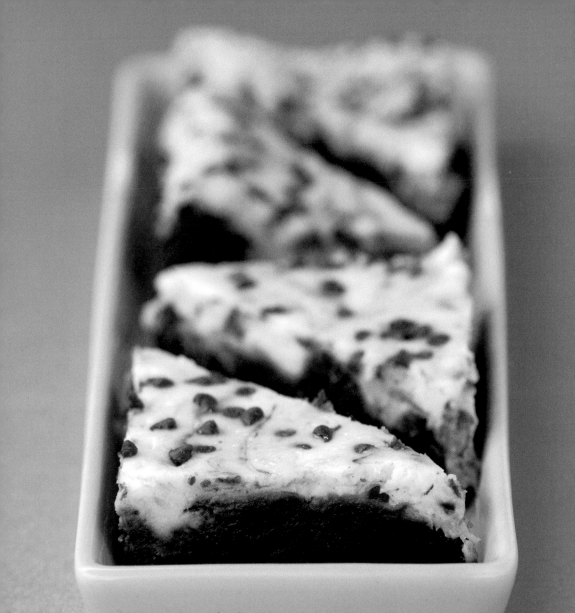

Chocolate Chip Cream Cheese Brownies

regular disposable plastic knife, running it through the brownies, top to bottom, end to end. Store the brownies chilled and in a tightly covered container, letting them warm on the counter for 10 minutes prior to serving, if desired.

Morsels

For the best flavor and texture, use arrowroot powder in the cream cheese topping—don't substitute cornstarch.

PUMPKIN PIE BROWNIES

MAKES 8 BROWNIES

WHEN AUTUMN ROLLS AROUND your sweet tooth starts asking tough questions. Brownies? Or pumpkin? Pumpkin? Or brownies? Instead of having a sweet tooth mutiny, call a ceasefire with this luscious concoction: a brownie base with pumpkin in the batter and then pumpkin pie filling poured on top and baked together in perfect harmony. Studded with chocolate chips, this makes a perfect treat for Halloween.

FOR THE BROWNIE LAYER:

4 ounces bittersweet chocolate, melted
1 cup canned or pureed pumpkin (not pumpkin pie filling)
¾ cup sugar
¼ cup canola oil
1 teaspoon pure vanilla extract
¾ cup flour
¼ cup Dutch cocoa powder
1 tablespoon tapioca flour (or arrowroot powder or cornstarch)
¼ teaspoon baking soda
¼ teaspoon salt

FOR THE PUMPKIN LAYER:

¾ cup canned or pureed pumpkin
2 tablespoons tapioca flour (or use arrowroot powder or cornstarch)
½ cup nondairy milk
⅓ cup sugar
1 teaspoon pure vanilla extract
¼ teaspoon ground ginger
¼ teaspoon ground cinnamon
A pinch of ground nutmeg
A pinch of ground allspice

TO DECORATE:

A handful of chocolate chips

VEGAN COOKIES INVADE YOUR COOKIE JAR

Pumpkin Pie Brownies

1. Preheat oven to 350°F. Grease a 9-inch springform pan, or use a 9-inch square pan, preferably lined with parchment paper.

TO MAKE THE BROWNIE LAYER:

1. Melt the chocolate (see page 24).
2. In a large mixing bowl, mix together the pumpkin, sugar, oil, and vanilla. Sift in the flour, cocoa powder, tapioca flour, baking soda, and salt and stir to combine, then mix in the melted chocolate.

TO MAKE THE PUMPKIN LAYER:

1. Mix all the ingredients in a large mixing bowl and stir until thoroughly combined.

TO ASSEMBLE:

1. Use a spatula to spread the brownie layer mixture into the prepared baking pan, taking care to bring the batter to the edges of the pan. Pour the pumpkin layer over it, leaving a little room at the edges if you can. Bake for 30 minutes, until the pumpkin layer looks fairly firm (a little jiggling is okay) and has cracked at the edges a bit.

2. Let the brownies cool for 20 minutes and then transfer the pan to the fridge to set for at least an hour and a half. Once set, decorate with chocolate chips, slice into wedges, and serve.

Morsels

A 15- or 16-ounce can of pumpkin will equal the amount of pumpkin needed for this recipe.

LEMON BARS

FOR TOO LONG HAVE WE VEGANS had our faces pressed against the glass of the dessert case and longing for the sweet tartness of those shimmering lemon bars. Well, you can stop scaring the staff of that bakery and start enjoying lemon bars today.

FOR THE CRUST:
- 1¾ cups all-purpose flour
- ⅔ cup powdered sugar, plus extra to decorate the bars
- ¼ cup cornstarch
- 1 cup nonhydrogenated margarine

FOR THE FILLING:
- 3 tablespoons agar agar flakes
- 1⅓ cups water
- 1 tablespoon finely grated lemon zest (from two large lemons)
- ⅔ cup fresh lemon juice
- 3 tablespoons arrowroot powder
- 1¼ cups sugar
- ⅛ teaspoon turmeric
- ¼ cup soy milk

1. Preheat oven to 350°F. Lightly grease a 13 x 9-inch baking pan.

2. Pulse flour, powdered sugar, and cornstarch in a food processor. Add margarine in spoonfuls and blend, 8 to 10 seconds, then pulse until the mixture resembles coarse meal. Sprinkle the mixture into the prepared baking pan and press it firmly into an even layer with slightly raised sides to hold in the filling. Refrigerate for about 30 minutes and then bake for 40 minutes; remove the pan from the oven and let it cool. Meanwhile, prepare the filling.

3. In a sauce pot, soak the agar agar in the water for 15 minutes. Meanwhile, zest your lemons and squeeze your lemon juice. Mix the arrow-

root powder into the lemon juice to dissolve.

4. When the agar agar has been soaking for 15 minutes, turn the heat up and bring to a boil. Boil for about 10 minutes, or until the agar agar is completely dissolved. Add the sugar and turmeric and boil until dissolved, about 3 minutes. Lower the heat to medium and add the arrowroot powder mixture, then add the lemon zest and soy milk.

Whisk constantly until the mixture thickens, about 5 minutes. It should not be rapidly boiling, but a low bubbling is okay.

5. Pour the mixture into the prepared crust, let it cool for 20 minutes, and then refrigerate for at least 3 hours, until the filling is only slightly jiggly and set. Use a sifter or a fine mesh strainer to sprinkle the bars with powdered sugar. Slice into squares and serve.

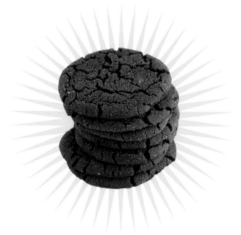

BIG FAT CRISPY RICE SQUARES

MAKES 9 HUGE SQUARES OR 12 SLIGHTLY SMALLER ONES

BIG, FAT CRISPY RICE SQUARES are found in better coffee shops all over the place these days, but common ingredients like gelatin-laced marshmallows and butter make these off-limits to vegans. Okay, there are also ultra-pristine animal-free ones, too, but usually they're too greasy or heavy with nut butters and raisins. What we really are craving is something more like the huge, crispy stacks from our childhood (and maybe yours, too!)

On that note, we're proud to present a crisp rice cereal treat that's huge, satisfying, yet still light, crunchy, and just sweet enough. We've eliminated the nut butter, kept the health nut–like addition of brown rice cereal, and enriched it with plenty of vanilla. A good firm pressing and freezing make these easy to slice. We also recommend making these in advance and letting them stand for a while (overnight is best), as these become sturdier given a little time to mellow. We like 'em plain, but perhaps try a fun little smattering of colorful sprinkles if you're in the mood to celebrate.

⅓ cup maple syrup
⅔ cup brown rice syrup
¼ cup nonhydrogenated margarine, cut into chunks
2½ teaspoons pure vanilla extract
¼ teaspoon almond, maple, or coconut extract
A pinch of salt
9 cups crispy brown rice cereal (one 10-ounce box of cereal)

1. Line an 8 x 8 x 3-inch square metal brownie pan with enough aluminum foil so that it folds over the sides of the pan by about an inch. Spray the bottom and sides of the covered pan with nonstick cooking spray.

2. In a large saucepan, combine the maple syrup and brown rice syrup; make sure to use a large pan with sides at least 4 inches tall, as the mixture will foam quite a bit when it boils. Stir over medium heat and

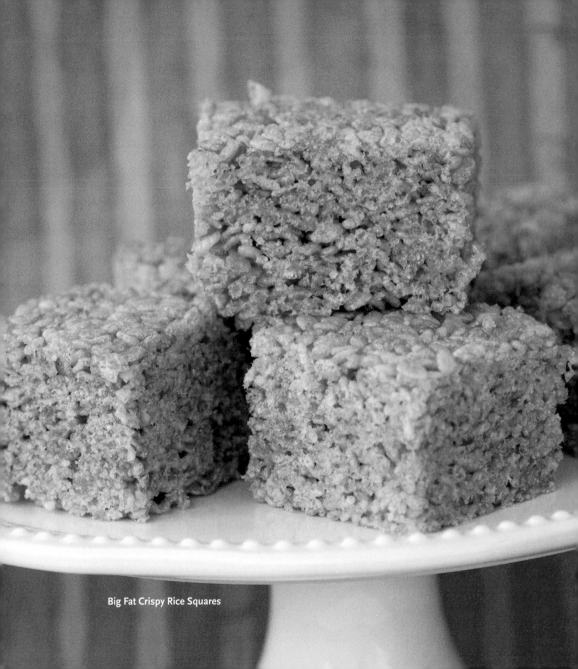

Big Fat Crispy Rice Squares

cook until the mixture comes to a full, rapid, foaming boil. Cook for 2 minutes, stirring constantly. Remove from heat, add the margarine, and stir until it's melted and mostly incorporated into syrup. Stir in the vanilla and almond extracts and salt.

3. Pour the cereal into a very large mixing bowl. Pour the cooked syrup mixture over the cereal, then use a large rubber spatula to stir and coat the cereal with the syrup mixture. Stir and fold for about 2 minutes, taking care to completely coat all of the cereal with syrup; the mixture should be very sticky. Use the spatula to scoop the coated cereal into the foil-lined pan, pushing the mixture around so that it's evenly distributed throughout the pan. It should heap somewhat over the top of the pan.

4. Tear a piece of waxed paper or parchment paper slightly larger than the size of the pan. Place the paper on top of the cereal mixture, then with your hands, firmly press down and mash the cereal so that it's now level with the edges of the pan. Evenly press all of the cereal down; this step is very important as it will help the crispy rice stick together, so make sure to keep pressing down firmly and evenly on the rice, even crushing it a little if necessary. When the cereal seems as level and firm as it's going to get, place the pan in the freezer and freeze for at least 2 hours or until very solid.

5. To slice, remove the pan from the freezer and slice immediately. The easiest way to do so is grab the edges of the foil, lift the entire contents out of pan, and flip it, wax paper side down, onto a cutting board. Peel off the foil from the top. Use a very sharp and heavy knife to slice the mixture into nine large squares or twelve smaller ones. For sturdier treats, loosely cover the squares and store in a cool place for 8 hours before serving. Frozen crispy rice squares can also be served right after slicing but may become slightly crumbly as they warm to room temperature.

FANCY COOKIES

FANCY MAY BE THE LEAST EASILY DEFINABLE QUALIFICATION of a cookie. Perhaps we like to label "fancy" any cookie that requires a more than just casually dropping or rolling out some dough onto a baking sheet. But maybe it's because these cookies—homemade vegan copycat "Oreos," frosted whiskey delights, hazelnut puffs sandwiched with chocolate truffle crème—make normal cookie eating into an occasion. No matter if you're dressed in a tux or in a track suit, you'll never feel like a plain Jane (or Joe) serving up any of these lovelies to friends or soon-to-be-friends.

Holiday cookie bakers, we've got your back, too, with bite-size fruitcake bars, powdery snowball-like wonders, and so many more that your family might start making up holidays just to ask for your specialty cookies on a regular basis.

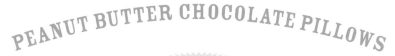

PEANUT BUTTER CHOCOLATE PILLOWS

MAKES 2 DOZEN COOKIES

CHOCOLATE-WITH-PEANUT-BUTTER DEVOTEES will totally stalk you once they bite into these seemingly ordinary chocolate cookies with a hidden peanut butter center. Or consider these a peanut butter ball with a chocolate cookie shell, and looking something like a plump round ravioli. Or a pillow, but edible, like the name says. Impatience is rewarded here: just a few minutes out of the oven, these cookies are dynamite—all warm and oozy inside. You can either press them down a little to give them a flattened shape, or leave the balls to flatten slightly on their own during baking.

FOR THE CHOCOLATE DOUGH:
- ½ cup canola oil
- 1 cup sugar
- ¼ cup pure maple syrup
- 3 tablespoons nondairy milk
- ½ teaspoon pure vanilla extract
- 1½ cups all-purpose flour
- ⅓ cup unsweetened cocoa powder
- 2 tablespoons black unsweetened cocoa powder or more regular unsweetened cocoa powder
- ½ teaspoon baking soda
- ¼ teaspoon salt

FOR THE FILLING:
- ¾ cup natural salted peanut butter, crunchy or creamy style
- ⅔ cup powdered sugar
- 2 to 3 tablespoons soy creamer or nondairy milk
- ¼ teaspoon pure vanilla extract

1. In a large mixing bowl, combine oil, sugar, maple syrup, nondairy milk, and vanilla and mix until smooth. Sift in flour, cocoa powder, black cocoa powder if using, baking soda, and salt. Mix to form a moist dough.

2. Make the peanut butter filling: In another mixing bowl, use a hand mixer to beat together peanut butter, powdered sugar, 2 tablespoons of the soy creamer, and vanilla to

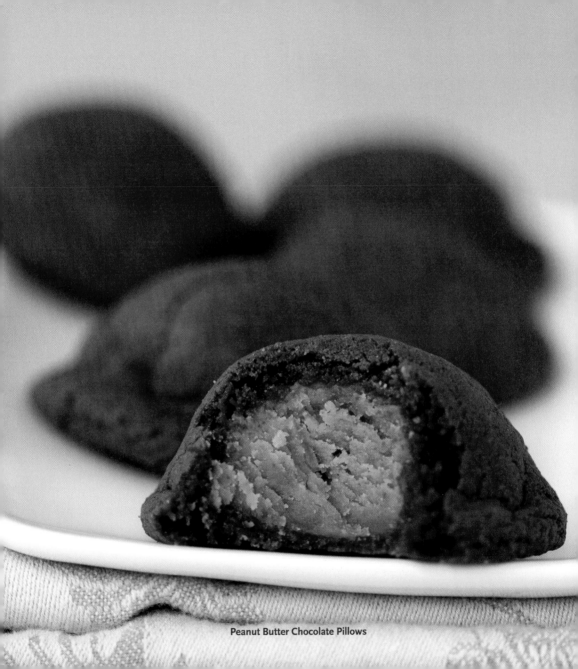

Peanut Butter Chocolate Pillows

form a moist but firm dough. If peanut butter dough is dry and crumbly (natural peanut butters have varying moisture contents), stir in the remaining tablespoon of nondairy milk. If dough is too wet knead in a little extra powdered sugar.

3. Preheat oven to 350°F. Line two baking sheets with parchment paper.

SHAPE THE COOKIES:

1. Create the centers of the cookies by rolling the peanut butter dough into twenty-four balls (try dividing dough in half, then each part in half again and roll each portion into six balls). Scoop a generous tablespoon of chocolate dough, flatten into a thin disc, and place a peanut butter ball in the center. Fold the sides of the chocolate dough up and around the peanut butter center and roll into a smooth ball between your palms. Place on a sheet of waxed paper and repeat with remaining dough. If desired, gently flatten cookies slightly, but this is not necessary.

2. Place the dough balls on lined baking sheets about 2 inches apart and bake for 10 minutes. Remove the sheet from the oven and let the cookies stand for 5 minutes before moving them to wire racks to complete cooling. Store cookies in tightly covered container. If desired, warm cookies in a microwave for 10 to 12 seconds before serving.

Morsels

If unsalted peanut butter is all you have, be sure add ¼ to ½ teaspoon salt to the peanut butter mixture.

MINONOS

FOR THOSE OF US WHO MISS suckling at the corporate teat of Pepperidge Farm, here is a veganized version of everyone's favorite chocolate sandwich cookie, the Milano. Even though there is a bit of orange zest in the batter, these aren't orange flavored, the zest just kind of pulls everything together and gives a sunny note of somethin' somethin'. We think bittersweet chocolate gives the most authentic flavor, but use semisweet if that's what you've got. And heed the directions to flour your hands before forming each cookie—otherwise the dough will stick.

⅓ cup nondairy milk
¾ cup sugar
½ cup canola oil
2 teaspoons pure vanilla extract
A scant 1 teaspoon finely grated orange zest
2 cups flour
2 tablespoons cornstarch
1 teaspoon baking powder
¼ teaspoon salt
6 ounces bittersweet or semisweet chocolate, chopped (or use chocolate chips)

1. Preheat oven to 350°F. Grease two large cookie sheets.

2. In a large mixing bowl, use a strong fork to mix together the nondairy milk, sugar, oil, vanilla, and zest. Add half the flour, along with the cornstarch, baking powder, and salt; mix well. Add the remaining flour and mix until you have a soft, pliable dough.

3. Make sure your hands are very clean and dry and dust them with flour. Stuff's about to get messy. Sort of.

4. Grab about 1 tablespoon's worth of dough and roll it into a ball, and then roll it into a log that's about

150   VEGAN COOKIES INVADE YOUR COOKIE JAR

1½ inches long. Flatten it with the palms of your hands to create an oval that is 2 inches long and 1 inch across, then straighten the edges out with your fingers. Basically, if you know what a Milano looks like, that's the shape you're going for. But this is homemade, so don't try to be perfect. You aren't a machine (or are you?).

5. Continue with the rest of the dough, flouring your hands before you form each cookie, until you have 16 cookies placed about 1 inch apart (they don't spread much.)

6. Bake the cookies for 14 to 16 minutes, until the tops are firm and the edges are ever-so-slightly browned. Remove the cookies from the oven and let them rest for 2 minutes. Use a thin, flexible spatula to transfer them to wire racks. Meanwhile, bake your next batch and melt your chocolate (page 24).

7. Once cookies are cool enough to handle (only about 10 minutes), take a cookie and dip the bottom into the chocolate. Then take another cookie and dip it, and place the dipped sides together to form a sandwich. Don't press them hard lest the chocolate smoosh out. Place the cookies on a tray or plate that will fit in your fridge. Continue with the remaining cookies until you have 16 sandwiches. Have a wet rag at the ready to wipe your fingers between putting the cookies together, to avoid chocolate fingerprints on the cookies. Or just lick the chocolate off. Or just decide that who cares about chocolate fingerprints.

8. Chill the cookies in the fridge to set for at least an hour. Bring them back to room temperature before serving (about ½ hour). Call it a day.

Cranberry Walnut
Thumbprints

CRANBERRY WALNUT THUMBPRINTS

MAKES 2 DOZEN COOKIES

FOR THE LOVE OF FALL, it's high time for a cookie that uses cranberry sauce. If a pretty maple-flavored thumbprint-style cookie ringed with walnuts and topped with sweet-tart cranberries doesn't get you into an autumnal mood then we don't know what will.

½ cup canola oil
¾ cup sugar
⅓ cup brown sugar
¼ cup nondairy milk
1½ teaspoons pure vanilla extract
½ teaspoon maple extract
1⅔ cups all-purpose flour
¼ cup cornstarch
1 teaspoon baking powder
½ teaspoon ground cinnamon
¼ teaspoon salt
1¼ cups finely chopped walnuts
1 cup jellied cranberry sauce, stirred till smooth

1. Preheat oven to 350°F. Line two baking sheets with parchment paper.

2. In a large bowl, beat together the oil, sugar, brown sugar, nondairy milk, and vanilla and maple extracts. Sift in the flour, cornstarch, baking powder, cinnamon, and salt. Stir to form a thick, stiff dough. If the dough seems too dry, add a tablespoon or so of nondairy milk.

3. Pour the chopped walnuts into a shallow bowl. Scoop the dough with a tablespoon and roll into balls, then roll the balls in the chopped walnuts and place them on the baking sheets, about 1 inch apart. Using the opposite end of a wooden spoon (the stick end), gen-

tly shape a hole into the center of each ball. (Hold the ball as you do this, as the dough may be fragile.) Pour a generous teaspoon of cranberry sauce or jam into each center. Bake for 16 to 18 minutes until the cranberry sauce seems mostly dry and cookies are firm. Allow the cookies to cool at least 5 minutes before carefully moving them to wire racks to complete cooling.

✳ *Morsels* ✳

Whole cranberry sauce makes these cookies even more three-dimensional. Cranberry sauce also contains more water than regular fruit preserves, hence the slightly longer baking time. Canned cranberry sauce works just fine here. If you don't like cranberries and would rather use your favorite red fruit preserve, cut the baking time down a minute or two.

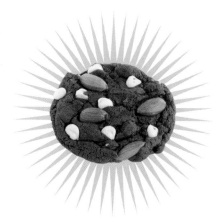

IRISH CREME KISSES

A BOUNTY OF WHISKEY, WALNUTS, COCOA, AND COFFEE AWAITS. This decadent cookie presents an adult-ish way to relish a heaping dollop of icing topped with chocolate curls. We should probably mention the frosting is boozalicious, too, so keep the kids clear of licking the frosting bowl for this one. Spirit-infused cookies like these taste even better the next day, so consider making 'em the night before your party. Plus the icing will firm up and make transporting these a little easier.

¼ cup nondairy milk
½ cup sugar
½ cup dark brown sugar
1 tablespoon ground flax seeds
¼ cup Irish whiskey
⅓ cup canola oil
4 teaspoons espresso powder
1½ teaspoons pure vanilla extract
¼ teaspoon almond extract
1½ cups all-purpose flour
2 tablespoons cornstarch
2 tablespoons cocoa powder
½ teaspoon baking powder
½ teaspoon baking soda
¼ teaspoon salt
1 cup finely chopped walnuts

FOR THE FROSTING:
2 tablespoons nonhydrogenated margarine, softened
1½ cups powdered sugar, sifted
1 tablespoon nondairy milk
2 to 3 teaspoons Irish whiskey
½ teaspoon pure vanilla extract

FOR SPRINKLING:
1 ounce dark semisweet chocolate, in bar form, at room temperature.

1. Preheat oven to 350°F. Line two baking sheets with parchment paper.
2. In a large mixing bowl, stir together the nondairy milk, sugar, brown

sugar, and flax seeds until smooth. Mix in the whiskey, oil, espresso powder, and vanilla and almond extracts. Sift in the all-purpose flour, cornstarch, cocoa powder, baking powder, baking soda, and salt. Mix to form a moist and somewhat sticky dough, then fold in the chopped walnuts.

3. Drop generously rounded tablespoons of dough 2 inches apart onto lined baking sheets. Bake for 12 to 14 minutes or until firm when pressed.

4. Let the cookies cool on the baking sheet for 5 minutes, then transfer them to wire racks to cool completely.

5. Make the frosting: In a large bowl, use a fork to combine the margarine with the powdered sugar until the mixture is crumbly. Stir in the nondairy milk, 2 teaspoons of the whiskey, and the vanilla and continue to stir to form a creamy, smooth frosting. If the mixture is too dry, add another teaspoon or more of whiskey; if too runny, sift in a tablespoon of powdered sugar. The frosting should be thick yet easy to spread.

6. Make the chocolate curls: Use a vegetable peeler and run it along the narrow edge of the bar to form small curls or flakes of chocolate. The chocolate should be soft enough so that curls form smoothly. You won't need very much, less than half a teaspoon per cookie should suffice.

7. Decorate the cookies by spreading a generous teaspoon of frosting onto the centers of the completely cooled cookies. Concentrate the frosting in the middle; do not spread to the edges. Sprinkle the chocolate curls onto the moist frosting and allow the cookies to set for about 30 minutes. If desired, chill the cookies to speed up the process. Store in a tightly covered container in a cool place.

NUTTY WEDDING COOKIES

MAKES ABOUT 2 DOZEN COOKIES

MEXICANS. ITALIANS. DANES. What do they have in common? Weddings! And these cookies! Here are those delicate, powder puff–looking, nut-laced shortbread cookies of many an ethnic name pertaining to matrimony. Because of all the powdered sugar, we don't recommend eating these while wearing black, so you may want to consider some other cookie for your goth wedding.

FOR COATING COOKIES:
- 1½ to 2 cups powdered sugar
- ½ cup nonhydrogenated margarine
- ½ cup nonhydrogenated vegetable shortening
- ⅔ cup powdered sugar
- 2 teaspoons pure vanilla extract
- ¼ teaspoon salt
- 1 tablespoon nondairy milk
- 1¾ cups all-purpose flour
- 1 cup finely ground pecans (about 4 ounces pecan halves; pulse with a food processor until finely ground)

1. Preheat oven to 325°F. Line two medium-size baking sheets with parchment paper.
2. Sift the powdered sugar that will be used for coating cookies onto a large plate, preferably one with a raised edge. Set aside.
3. In a large bowl, with a hand mixer, beat together the margarine and shortening until light and creamy. Beat in the powdered sugar until smooth. Add the vanilla, salt, nondairy milk, and half the flour and beat until ingredients are moistened. Add the remaining flour and the pecans. Beat on high speed for 3 to 5 minutes to form a soft and fluffy dough. If the dough appears crumbly, don't fret, just keep beating the dough until it becomes moist enough to stick together when pressed into a ball.

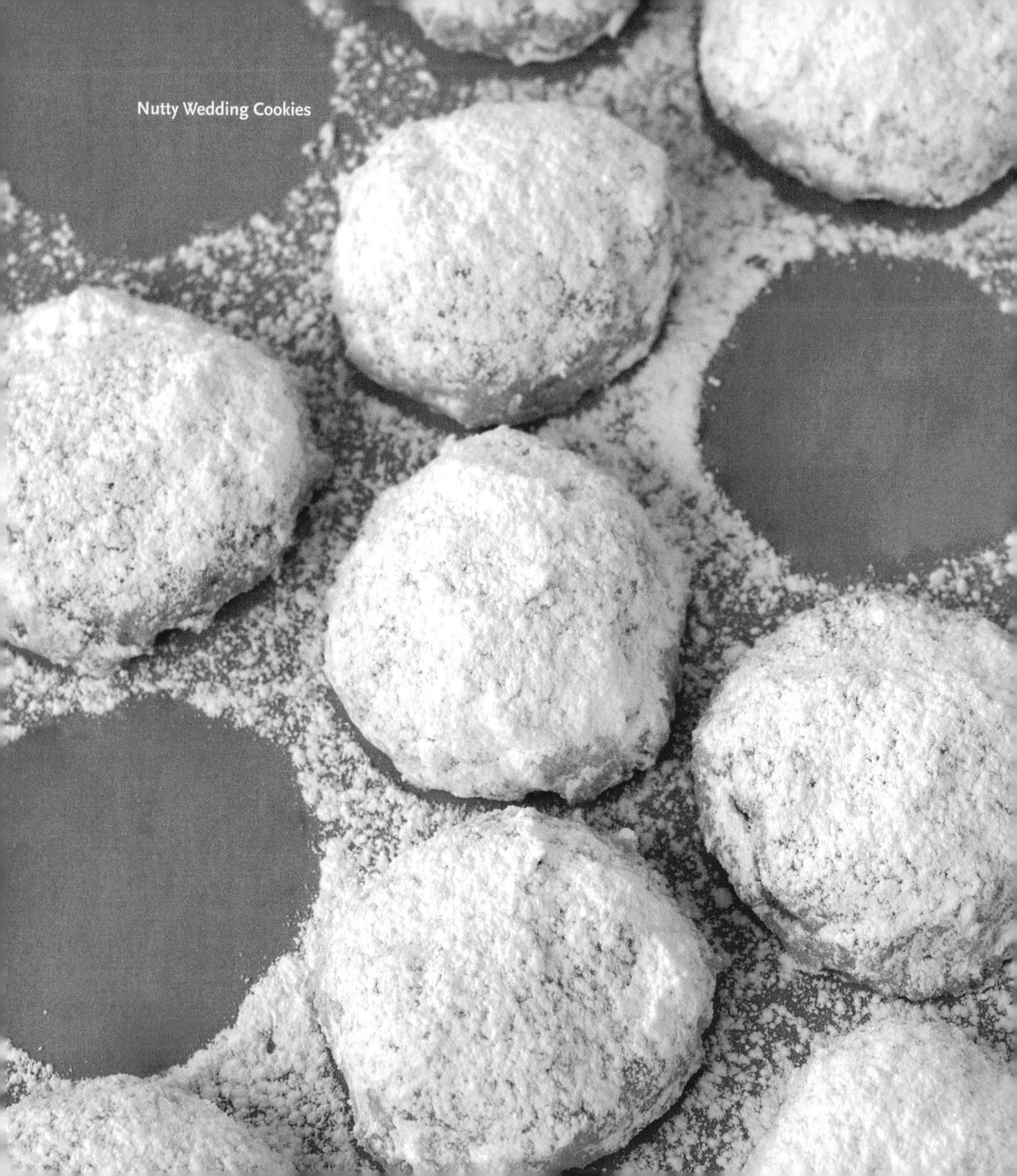

4. For each cookie, scoop a generous tablespoon of dough and roll it into a ball. Place balls of dough 2 inches apart on lined baking sheets. Bake for 14 to 18 minutes, until the edges just begin to brown. Remove the cookies from the oven and let them cool on the cookie sheet for 8 minutes. While the cookies are still warm move 2 to 3 cookies to the dish with the sifted powdered sugar. Carefully turn cookies several times to form a thick coating of powdered sugar. Very gently tap off excess sugar and place the cookies on wire racks to finish cooling. Repeat with the remaining warm cookies. Store in a tightly covered container. These cookies are best eaten the day they are baked, preferably within a few hours. See note about refreshing the powdered sugar coating if serving cookies later or, if you must, the next day.

Variation

ALMOND WEDDINGS: Substitute 4 ounces of sliced almonds for pecans. Pulse in a food processor until finely ground.

❋ Morsels ❋

✦ Coating the warm cookies in powdered sugar can sometimes leave an uneven surface, especially if the cookies sit for more than a day or have been transported. For a pretty and evenly coated top, sift a little extra powdered sugar on the cookies when they're absolutely finished cooling, preferably just before serving them.

✦ Place a sheet of waxed paper underneath the wire cooling rack to catch excess powdered sugar and make clean-up all the easier.

NYC Black and White Cookies

NYC BLACK AND WHITE COOKIES

MAKES 16 LARGE COOKIES

LOOKING OUT AT YOU LIKE A SULTRY, HEAVY-LIDDED EYE from many a bakery window, these large, cakey cookies are an NYC fixture. Don't know black and white cookies? Imagine not quite a cookie but a slightly domed mini-cake (a drop cake, technically), flipped over onto its back then painted half chocolate, half vanilla—with sugary-sweet royal icing and fudgy icing. Unfortunately, because they're commonplace, one can't always vouch for freshness or quality. And likely they're not vegan anyway. So instead, why not make a batch at home and you'll be assured of super-freshness and veganitude, yay!

1 cup soy milk
2 teaspoons lemon juice
½ cup canola or safflower oil
1¼ cups sugar
1½ teaspoons pure vanilla extract
¼ teaspoon lemon extract or ½
   teaspoon finely grated lemon zest
¼ teaspoon orange extract or ½
   teaspoon finely grated orange zest
2½ cups all-purpose flour
¼ cup cornstarch
1¼ teaspoons baking powder
½ teaspoon baking soda
¾ teaspoon salt

FOR THE ICINGS:
3½ to 4 cups powdered sugar
¼ cup boiling water (plus several
   additional tablespoons of hot water)
1 to 2 drops vanilla or almond extract,
   optional
⅔ cup semisweet chocolate chips

1. Preheat oven to 350°F. Line two baking sheets with parchment paper.
2. In a medium bowl, combine the soy milk and lemon juice; allow the mixture to sit 1 minute to curdle. Add the oil, sugar, vanilla, and

lemon and orange extracts and whisk until well blended.

3. In a large bowl, sift together the flour, cornstarch, baking powder, baking soda, and salt. Form a well in the center of the flour mixture and pour in the soy milk mixture. Stir to combine, taking care to moisten the flour at the bottom of the bowl. Stir until almost all of the lumps have dissolved and a very thick batter forms.

4. With an ice-cream scoop or ¼ cup measuring cup (you can use a ⅓ cup measuring cup for big, bakery-size cookies), scoop the batter onto the baking sheets, leaving 3 inches of space between cookies. These cookies will spread so leave adequate room between them. Bake for 18 to 20 minutes, till a toothpick inserted into the center of a cookie comes out clean. Remove the cookies from the oven, allow them to cool 2 minutes, then carefully remove them from the parchment paper. Flip the cookies upside down and place them on wire racks to complete cooling.

5. When all the cookies are done baking, prepare the white icing. Scoop the powdered sugar into a large metal bowl. Add ¼ cup boiling water and stir vigorously with a wire whisk. Add a drop of vanilla or almond extract if desired. If necessary, dribble in additional hot water by the tablespoon till a glossy, thin-but-spreadable icing forms. If it's too runny whisk in a little bit of extra powdered sugar.

6. Dust any crumbs off the flat bottoms of cookies. With a frosting spatula, scoop some icing onto the flat side (the former bottom) of each cookie and spread an even, not-too-thick but opaque layer of frosting to the edges. Use the edge of the spatula to scrape away any extra icing dripping off the sides. Return cookies to cooling racks to allow the iced tops of the cookies to dry enough so surface feels set and not sticky. You will have some extra icing remaining (about ½ cup) that you'll be using to make the chocolate icing.

7. While the white icing is drying, prepare the chocolate icing. In a double boiler or microwave, melt the chocolate chips (page 24) until smooth. Add the melted chocolate to the leftover white icing and use a wire whisk to blend it until thick, smooth, and glossy. It should be slightly thicker than the white icing. If the chocolate icing is too thick or grainy, stir in very hot water, 1 tablespoon at a time, until the desired consistency is reached.

With the frosting spatula, ice one-half of each cookie over the vanilla icing. Feel free to layer it on thickly just because it's chocolate icing. Return the cookies to the wire racks to set the frosted tops until they feel dry to the touch.

8. NYC Black and White Cookies are best eaten the day they're made. If that's not possible, store them in a tightly covered container in a cool place.

Morsels

This dough resembles a very thick sticky cake batter, so no skipping lining the baking sheets with parchment paper. For best results, scoop batter with an ice-cream scoop (the kind with a release trigger); dip it occasionally in water to ensure easier dough dropping. This recipe makes over a dozen large, palm-size cookies, but when shaping dough try a tablespoon or mini ice cream scoop to make lots of small 'n' cute.

SWEET CHOCOLATE PRETZELS

MAKES 2 DOZEN COOKIES

A SIMPLE, CHOCOLATY, BUTTERY COOKIE in a fun pretzel shape that's popular with the crafty cookie set and fans of food that's shaped like one thing and tastes like another. And an unexpected way to rock the holiday cookie tray. Pearl sugar—large snow-white nuggets of crunchy sugar—makes them really pop, but regular decorating sugar looks spiffy, too.

Look for pearl sugar in baking supply shops that specialize in fancy stuff or European baking ingredients. Large, uncolored crystal decorator sugar is a good stand-in for pearl sugar and looks sneakily like actual pretzel salt.

½ cup nonhydrogenated margarine, softened
⅓ cup sugar
⅓ cup brown sugar
1½ teaspoons pure vanilla extract
A generous pinch of salt
⅓ cup nondairy milk
⅓ cup unsweetened cocoa powder
2 tablespoons black cocoa powder
1⅔ cups all-purpose flour
3 tablespoons sweetened soy creamer or nondairy milk for brushing
2 to 3 tablespoons pearl sugar or large crystal decorator sugar for sprinkling

1. Preheat oven to 350°F. Line two baking sheets with parchment paper.

2. In a large mixing bowl, use a hand mixer to cream together the margarine, sugar, brown sugar, vanilla, and salt until fluffy, scraping down the sides of the bowl frequently with a rubber spatula. Beat in the nondairy milk until smooth, then sift in the natural cocoa powder, black cocoa powder, and all-purpose flour. Mix to form a firm yet slightly moist dough.

3. Knead the dough a few times and divide into four equal balls. If the dough feels too sticky, very lightly dust a little flour onto your hands and the work surface, but try not to use too much flour. The dough should be moist enough to be easily pliable and not overly prone to cracking.

4. Divide a ball into six pieces. Gently roll each piece into a 6- to 8-inch rope, pinching in any cracks that may form. Bend each rope into a pretzel shape (consult an actual pretzel if you're feeling flummoxed) and gently press down to secure the shape. Slide a thin metal spatula under each pretzel and move 'em to the prepared baking sheet, spacing them about 1 inch apart. Repeat with remaining dough.

5. Brush each pretzel with soy creamer and sprinkle with pearl or decorator sugar. Bake for 10 to 12 minutes until cookies are firm.

6. Let the cookies cool on the baking sheet for 5 minutes, then transfer them to wire racks to cool completely. Store in a tightly covered container.

Morsels
No black cocoa powder? Substitute more cocoa powder.

Starry Fudge Shortbread

STARRY FUDGE SHORTBREAD

MAKES 2-1/2 DOZEN OR MORE COOKIES

THANKS STELLA. We've had a crush on your "Swiss" cookies forever but we've learned to live without. But now with a pastry bag and a dream, it's simple to make at home buttery little piped cookies crowned with a chocolaty ganache center. Use quality semisweet chocolate for the filling and you'll have some class-act cookies that will run circles 'round the store-bought stuff.

You'll need a large pastry bag fitted with a jumbo star tip (look for size number 827, or a very large tip with an opening around 1/2-inch wide) to pipe out stars of dough. A spritz cookie press fitted with a star mold can be used, but you may find pastry bags and tips easier to handle (plus they involve minimal investment and are easy enough to find at baking supply stores or online). These cuties are a wee bit more labor-intensive than typical shortbread but fun to make, with yummy results.

This dough is also excellent for making traditional holiday spritz cookies. Use your favorite flavor extracts, bring out the wreath and Christmas-tree shaped cookie nozzles, and your GINGERBREAD CUT-OUT COOKIES (page 226) will need to make room on the cookie plate come holiday season.

FOR THE SHORTBREAD COOKIES:
- 1 cup nonhydrogenated margarine, softened
- ⅔ cup sugar
- A pinch of salt
- 2 teaspoons pure vanilla extract
- ¾ teaspoon almond extract
- 2 cups all-purpose flour
- ¼ cup cornstarch
- ¼ cup nondairy milk

FOR THE CHOCOLATE GANACHE FILLING:
- ¼ cup nondairy milk
- 1 tablespoon maple syrup
- 4 ounces semisweet vegan chocolate (either chopped or chips)
- A few extra teaspoons of nondairy milk to use for shaping cookies

1. Preheat oven to 350°F. Have ready two ungreased, nonstick baking sheets. Avoid using parchment paper or greasing the sheet as this cookie dough requires a little bit of "grip" when it's piped onto a baking surface.

2. In a large bowl, use a hand mixer to beat the margarine, sugar, and salt until light and fluffy, about 5 minutes. Scrape the sides of the bowl frequently. Add the vanilla and almond extracts and beat to combine. In a separate bowl, sift together the flour and cornstarch. Add half the flour mixture to the margarine mixture, first folding in the flour with a spatula so that it doesn't fly all over the place when using the mixer beaters. Beat until the flour is mostly combined and add the rest of the flour, using the spatula as before. Mixture may be a little crumbly. Beat in the nondairy milk to form a soft dough.

3. Fit a jumbo (number 827 or ½-inch-wide opening) star pastry tip into your pastry bag and load it about halfway full. Hold the edges of the bag and shake it a few times to help push the dough further down toward the nozzle. Use one hand to twist down the end of the bag until dough begins to press out of the tip, and with your other hand, guide the nozzle onto the baking sheet. Pipe stars of dough 1½ to 1¾ inches wide and about 2 inches apart onto the baking sheet. To remove the nozzle from freshly pressed cookie dough, gently twist and pull the nozzle away from the cookie.

4. After you're finished piping out the cookies, use the back of a teaspoon (the circular kind used for measuring is best) or your finger to create the indentations into the cookies that will eventually hold the melted ganache. First dip the back of the teaspoon in nondairy milk, then press it into the center of the dough star. Gently move it around a little to create a well at least ¼ inch deep, taking care not to press a hole into the bottom of the cookie. The wider the well the more ganache it can contain!

5. Bake the cookies for 12 minutes until puffed and the edges are just starting to turn golden. After baking, if some of the wells look too puffed, gently press the hot cookie centers again with the back of the measuring teaspoon. Let the cookies cool on the baking sheet for 5 minutes before using a thin spatula to move them to wire racks to complete cooling.

6. While cookies are baking, make the chocolate ganache. In a small saucepan over medium-high heat, bring the nondairy milk and maple syrup to a gentle boil. Immediately remove from heat and add chocolate. Use a silicon spatula to stir the chocolate into the nondairy milk mixture. Keep stirring until chocolate is completely melted and very smooth, about 6 to 8 minutes. Allow the ganache to cool about 10 minutes before proceeding. It should thicken slightly but still remain pourable.

7. Cookies can be filled with ganache while still warm or after they are cooled. Spoon ½ to 1 teaspoon of warm (not hot) ganache carefully into centers, filling each as much as possible but taking care not to overflow. Allow the ganache to cool at least an hour or more to completely set. If desired, chill the cookies to speed up the process. Store in a tightly covered container in a cool location.

Variations

CHERRY STAR COOKIES: Omit the ganache, press half a candied cherry into the center of cookies before baking, and there you have that bakery classic: the candied-cherry shortbread star cookie.

Morsels

Allow the ganache centers of these cookies at least an hour to firm up. To help speed the process chill the cookies for at least 20 minutes. Chilled ganache will have a clouded appearance; allow the cookies to sit at room temperature for 5 minutes for the chocolate surface shine to return.

SPRITZ COOKIES: Use this dough in your cookie press fitted with your favorite spritz design plates. Depending on how big your press is, you can expect anywhere from 3 to 5 dozen cookies. For even more festive cookies, try flavoring the dough with extracts (citrus, fruit, or anise) and sprinkling the unbaked cookies with colored decorating sugar. If your cookies are very small (under 1½ inches) you may need to reduce the baking time by 2 to 4 minutes.

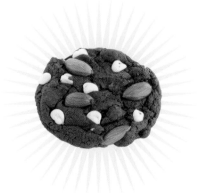

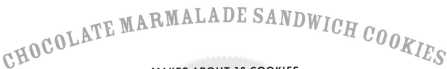

CHOCOLATE MARMALADE SANDWICH COOKIES

FOR THE CHOCOLATE-AND-ORANGE LOVER IN YOUR LIFE. Orange marmalade sandwiched in dark chocolaty wafer cookies laced with orange zest. These look best if you use the lintzertorte-style cookie cutters, so that a window of marmalade peeks through to entice them into a sinful world of orangey goodness.

⅔ cup sugar
¼ cup oil
¼ cup nondairy milk
1 tablespoon grated orange zest
1 teaspoon vanilla
1 cup all-purpose flour
½ cup Dutch cocoa powder
1 tablespoon cornstarch
½ teaspoon baking powder
¼ teaspoon salt
⅓ to ½ cup orange marmalade
A few tablespoons powdered sugar
    (optional)

1. In a mixing bowl, vigorously mix the sugar, oil, and nondairy milk. Mix in the zest and vanilla.
2. Sift in flour, cocoa powder, cornstarch, baking powder, and salt. Mix until well combined. The dough should be stiff but pliable. Divide in half and form into two large discs; flatten the discs and refrigerate them for about an hour.
3. Preheat oven to 350°F. Line two cookie sheets with parchment paper. Roll the dough out about ⅛ inch thick onto a lightly floured surface. Use a 1½- to 2-inch cookie cutter to make circles. Transfer the cookies to baking sheets with a thin spatula. Roll the dough scraps out to get a few more cookies.
4. Bake the cookies for 7 minutes. Let them cool on baking sheets for 2 minutes before moving them to wire racks to cool completely.

5. Once cool, spread about a teaspoon of marmalade onto one cookie and sandwich it with another cookie. Sprinkle with sifted powdered sugar if desired. (The sugar that falls on the marmalade will dissolve.) Store in a tightly sealed container.

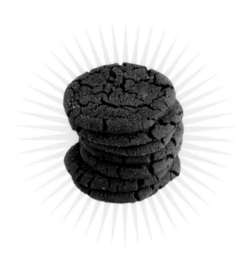

LAZY SAMOAS®
(Toasted Coconut Chocolate Cookies)

MAKES OVER 2 DOZEN COOKIES

A YUMMY, FUN-TO-MAKE, AND TOTALLY VEGAN ALTERNATIVE to the ever-popular Girl Scout favorites. We left out the fussy shortbread base in favor of even more toasted coconut and brown sugar cookie, but we kept the chocolate-dipped bottom and final drizzle of even more chocolate, essentially making them both more delicious and a little more lazy.

2 cups grated unsweetened coconut
⅓ cup unrefined coconut oil
¾ cup firmly packed brown sugar
⅓ cup nondairy milk
1 tablespoon ground flax seeds
1½ teaspoons pure vanilla extract
1 cup all-purpose flour
¼ teaspoon baking soda
½ teaspoon salt

FOR DECORATING:
1 cup chocolate chips
2 tablespoons unrefined coconut oil

1. Preheat oven to 350°F. Line two baking sheets with parchment paper.
2. Pour the grated coconut into a large heavy skillet and toast over medium-low heat. Stir occasionally and toast coconut to a light golden brown, about 8 to 10 minutes. Watch carefully to avoid burning. Promptly remove the coconut from the heat and stir it occasionally as it cools. If the coconut continues to turn overly brown promptly pour from skillet into a large dish and spread around to help hasten cooling and stop cooking.
3. In a large mixing bowl, combine the coconut oil, brown sugar, nondairy milk, flax seeds, and vanilla until well blended and smooth. Sift in the all-purpose flour, baking soda, and salt and mix to form a

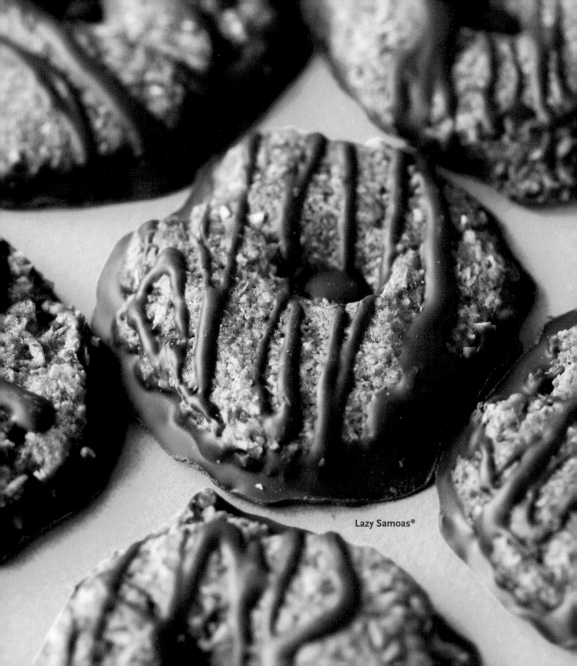
Lazy Samoas®

thick batter. Fold in the toasted coconut.

4. Scoop about 1 tablespoon of dough 2 inches apart onto the baking sheets. Flatten each cookie with the back of a measuring cup and use your fingertip to work a small hole into each center. Bake for 8 minutes, until the edges of the cookies are golden.

5. Let the cookies cool on the baking sheet for 5 minutes, then transfer them to wire racks to cool completely. Transfer the cooled cookies onto waxed paper, then place them onto a cutting board or other firm surface that can be easily slid onto a refrigerator shelf.

6. While cookies are cooling, melt chocolate chips in a microwave or double boiler (page 24), then stir the coconut oil into the melted chocolate. Allow the chocolate to cool for 5 minutes to thicken slightly. Dip cookie bottoms into the chocolate and return them to the waxed paper. Now drizzle the remaining chocolate over the cookies, either by dipping a fork into the melted chocolate or by pouring the chocolate into a pastry bag fitted with a very small round tip. Chill the cookies for at least 30 minutes to completely firm up the chocolate. Store the cookies in a loosely covered container in a very cool place.

Morsels

We love how unrefined coconut oil packs even more sweet, nutty coconut aroma and flavor into these little cookies.

HAZELNUT FUDGE DREAMIES

MAKES ABOUT 2 DOZEN SANDWICH COOKIES

CALLING THESE JUST SANDWICH COOKIES would be a shame. Such delicate little puffs of hazelnut shortbread joined by a schmear of chocolate truffle espresso fudge are better than just cookie sandwiches, they are like angels singing, unicorns prancing, and stuff like that. Enjoy these with strong coffee or after a fabuloso Italian meal. A nice addition to holiday cookie selections, too, but don't wait till then to try these!

FOR THE COOKIES:
- ½ cup nonhydrogenated margarine
- ½ cup nonhydrogenated vegetable shortening
- ¾ cup powdered sugar
- ¼ teaspoon salt
- 1 teaspoon pure vanilla extract
- 3 tablespoons hazelnut liqueur (see tip)
- 1⅔ cups all-purpose flour
- 1 cup finely ground toasted hazelnuts (about 1¼ cups whole nuts; measure, toast, then pulse with a food processor until finely ground)

FOR THE CHOCOLATE GANACHE FILLING:
- ⅓ cup nondairy milk
- 2 teaspoons instant espresso powder
- 1 tablespoon nonhydrogenated margarine
- 1¼ cups semisweet chocolate chips
- 1 tablespoon hazelnut liqueur

1. Preheat oven to 350°F. Line two baking sheets with parchment paper.
2. In a large mixing bowl, use a hand mixer to beat together the margarine, shortening, powdered sugar, and salt until fluffy and creamy, about 2 minutes. Use a rubber spatula to scrape down the dough from the sides of the bowl occasionally. Beat in the vanilla and hazelnut liqueur, then sift in the flour and add the hazelnuts. Combine to form a soft, thick dough. If the

dough seems a little sticky, chill it for 10 to 15 minutes to firm, but this step is not necessary to proceed with baking.

3. For each cookie, scoop 1 rounded teaspoon of dough, form it into a ball, and place the balls 1 inch apart on the baking sheets. Bake for 10 minutes, until the cookies are puffed and have slightly spread. Let the cookies cool on the baking sheet for 5 minutes, then transfer them to wire racks to cool completely.

4. While the cookies are cooling, make the chocolate ganache filling. In a small saucepan, bring the nondairy milk to a boil. Remove from heat, whisk in the espresso powder to dissolve, then immediately add the margarine and chocolate chips. Stir the mixture with a rubber spatula to melt the chips and margarine; continue to stir until chocolate has completely melted and is smooth and glossy. Stir in the hazelnut liqueur and set the mixture aside to cool for 10 min-

utes, then place it in the freezer for about 15 minutes to firm up. The mixture should be firm enough to spread but not completely hardened. Stir with a rubber spatula to make a spreadable consistency.

5. Spread the chocolate mixture generously on the underside of a cookie and sandwich with a second cookie. Both flat undersides should be facing the filling. Place sandwiched cookies on a platter, then move the platter to the refrigerator to firm the filling completely. Store in a tightly covered container in a cool place.

✳ *Morsels* ✳

✦ Leftover filling? Make real truffles! Roll chilled filling into bite-size balls and then roll in a little cocoa powder. Chill until firm and serve.

✦ Hazelnut liqueur, such as Frangelico, makes these special. If you want to use hazelnut extract instead, use 1½ teaspoons in the cookie dough plus 3 tablespoons nondairy milk. Use 1 teaspoon in the chocolate ganache filling.

NUTTER BETTERS SANDWICH COOKIES

MAKES 2-1/2 TO 3 DOZEN SANDWICH COOKIES,

depending on shape and size of cookie cutter

PRESENTING A PEANUT BUTTER SANDWICH COOKIE that's crunchy, creamy, and delivers all the peanut-buttery goodness your inner kiddie longs for. Molasses enhances the roasted peanut flavor and a touch of homemade oat flour adds an unexpected light, crisp finish to the cookie. The filling is a classic peanut-buttercream frosting, a little less sweet and more peanutty than "buttery."

In regards to the shape of your cookies, it's really up to you. As of this writing, finding an actual peanut-shaped cookie cutter has been a quest yielding few satisfying results. Slicing the dough into even little rectangular "fingers" doesn't require a cookie cutter but does require a ruler and some measuring skills (all of the cookies should be the same shape and size for effective sandwiches!). The easiest option just may be using your favorite 2- to 2-1/4-inch-wide circular cutter.

FOR THE PEANUT BUTTER COOKIES:
- ½ cup creamy natural peanut butter
- ½ cup nonhydrogenated vegetable shortening
- ½ cup sugar
- ½ cup dark brown sugar
- ¼ cup nondairy milk
- 1½ teaspoons pure vanilla extract
- ½ cup quick-cooking oats
- 2 cups all-purpose flour
- ½ teaspoon baking soda
- ¼ teaspoon salt

FOR THE PEANUT BUTTER CREME FILLING:
- ½ cup creamy natural peanut butter
- ¼ cup nonhydrogenated margarine, softened
- 2 teaspoons molasses (regular, not blackstrap)
- 1 teaspoon pure vanilla extract
- 1 cup powdered sugar, sifted
- 4 to 6 teaspoons nondairy creamer or nondairy milk
- A few teaspoons of sugar for sprinkling

PREPARE THE COOKIE DOUGH:

1. In a large bowl, cream the peanut butter, shortening, sugar, and dark brown sugar with electric beaters until light and fluffy, about 4 to 6 minutes. Use a rubber spatula to scrape down the sides of the bowl frequently. Beat in the nondairy milk and vanilla.

2. In a food processor, pulse the quick-cooking oats several times to form a coarse flour. Sift the all-purpose flour, baking soda, and salt into the peanut butter mixture, add the oat flour, and use a rubber spatula to fold the flour mixture into the moist ingredients a few times. Finish the mixing with a hand mixer, beating until a soft dough forms. If the dough appears a little dry or crumbly, beat in a little nondairy milk 1 tablespoon at a time until the dough is soft and nonsticky. Press the dough into a ball, flatten it to about 1½ inches thick, and wrap it in plastic wrap. Chill the dough for 30 minutes while preparing the filling and preheating the oven.

PREPARE THE PEANUT BUTTER FILLING:

1. In another large bowl, using a hand mixer, cream together the peanut butter and margarine until light and fluffy, about 3 minutes. Add the molasses and vanilla and beat to combine. Sift in the powdered sugar, then use a fork to combine the ingredients to moisten. Finish mixing with the hand mixer; the mixture should appear slightly crumbly. Drizzle in 4 teaspoons of nondairy creamer and beat until a thick yet creamy, frosting-like mass forms. If the filling still appears dry, drizzle in more nondairy milk by the teaspoon. The mixture should be thick but spreadable. If for some reason it gets too moist, beat in a tablespoon or two of sifted powdered sugar. Set the filling aside at room temperature.

SHAPE AND BAKE THE COOKIES:

1. Preheat oven to 350°F. Line two baking sheets with parchment paper. Have ready a rolling pin; a little all-purpose flour for dusting; cookie cutters; a clean fork; a clean,

wide surface for rolling dough; and a thin metal spatula for lifting the unbaked cookies onto the cookie sheet. Have ready those few teaspoons of sugar for sprinkling, too.

2. Lightly dust your work surface and rolling pin with flour. Slice the chilled dough in half, place one half back in the refrigerator, and form the other half into an oblong shape on the work surface, dusting it with flour as needed. Roll the dough to approximately ⅜-inch thick and sprinkle it lightly with sugar. Cut it into shapes and use the metal spatula to carefully lift the cookies onto the baking sheets, spacing them about 1 inch apart. If you are cutting the dough into rectangles, use a ruler to guide you and aim to cut the cookies 1 inch wide by 2½ to 2¾ inches long. Use a fork to gently poke holes halfway through the dough at random intervals to create a peanut shell–like texture. Be sure to cut an even number of cookies to have matching pairs for sand-

wiches. Repeat the rolling and cutting of cookies with the remaining dough.

3. Bake the cookies 10 to 12 minutes, until they are firm and the edges are just starting to turn golden. Cool the cookies on the baking sheet for 2 minutes before moving them to wire racks to complete cooling.

4. Assemble the sandwiches only after the cookies have completely cooled. Spread 1 to 1½ teaspoons of filling on a cookie, top with another cookie, and gently press down, taking care to have the top side of the top cookie facing upwards. These cookies look best with a generous amount of filling, so don't skimp. A useful filling technique is to mound the filling toward the center of the cookie while scraping the sides, so when the top cookie is pressed down the filling will bulge a little. Store in a tightly covered container in a cool place.

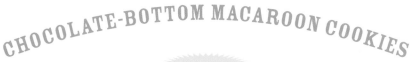

CHOCOLATE-BOTTOM MACAROON COOKIES

MAKES 2 DOZEN COOKIES

A CRISPY, COCONUTTY OUTSIDE AND A MOIST, SWEET INSIDE. That sounds good, right? Well, what if we told you it's also dipped in chocolate? These are irresistibly adorable morsels that look like they could be currency for magical forest creatures. A touch of almond extract really brings out the coconut. For variety, try the cocoa variation and have a double chocolate extravaganza.

3 ounces extra firm silken tofu, like Mori-Nu (¼ of the package)
⅓ cup canola oil
2 tablespoons nondairy milk
½ cup sugar
½ teaspoon almond extract
1 teaspoon pure vanilla extract
1 cup all-purpose flour
¾ teaspoon baking powder
¼ teaspoon salt
1½ cups unsweetened shredded coconut
½ cup chocolate chips, melted (page 24)

1. Preheat oven to 350°F. Line two baking sheets with parchment paper.

2. Puree the tofu, oil, and nondairy milk in a blender or food processor until smooth, scraping down the sides with a spatula to make sure you get everything. Transfer the mixture to a mixing bowl. Mix in the sugar and extracts. Mix in the flour, baking powder, and salt until well incorporated. Add the coconut and mix until a stiff dough forms.

3. Drop the cookies by the tablespoon onto the cookie sheets 2 inches apart from each other; they don't spread much at all. Don't smooth the tops out; it's cool if they have some pieces of coconut sticking out to get a little browned. Bake for 12 to 14 minutes. When ready, the bot-

toms should be lightly browned and the tops just barely flecked with color in a few spots.

4. Let the cookies cool on the sheets for 2 minutes or so, then transfer them to wire racks to cool completely. In the meantime, melt the chocolate. Line a cutting board with parchment paper (it's fine to reuse the stuff you lined the sheets with). When cookies have cooled completely, dip the bottoms in chocolate and set them, chocolate side down, on the parchment paper. Place the cookies in the fridge to set for at least 15 minutes. Store in a tightly sealed container at room temperature. If it's hot out, keep them in the fridge so the chocolate doesn't melt.

Variations

COCOA MACAROON COOKIES: Replace ¼ cup of the flour with ¼ cup unsweetened cocoa.

CHIPPER MACAROON COOKIES: Fold 1 cup mini chocolate chips into the dough.

TOUCH OF ORANGE MACAROON COOKIES: Add 2 teaspoons orange zest to the wet ingredients, leave out the almond extract.

Or try any combination of variations above!

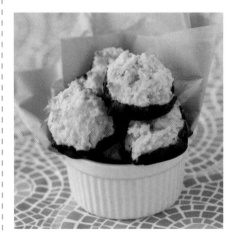

MACADAMIA LACE COOKIES

YOU KNOW WHEN YOU'RE DIGGING INTO A BOWL of vanilla bean ice cream and you're like, "This is nice but it could use a big caramel disc in it?" Well, here you are. Macadamia Laces are thin and pretty filigree cookies that are just perfect as fancy ice cream toppers, or enjoyed as caramelly treats on their own. Macadamias make these really buttery-tasting, yet they don't even have any margarine. We know times are tight, so if you need to sub blanched almonds, go for it. If you have a window in your oven these are fun to watch melt into the cookie sheet. You will be positive that they won't come out right, but they will! Just believe!

½ cup brown sugar, lightly packed

3 tablespoons canola oil

¼ cup pure maple syrup or agave nectar

1 tablespoon water

1 teaspoon pure vanilla extract

⅓ cup all-purpose flour

½ teaspoon cornstarch

⅛ teaspoon salt

½ cup roasted, unsalted macadamias, pulsed into coarse crumbs in a food processor (a few larger pieces are okay)

1. Preheat oven to 350°F. Line two baking sheets with parchment paper.

2. Combine sugar, oil, syrup, and water in a mixing bowl. Mix vigorously. Stir in the vanilla. Add the flour, cornstarch, and salt and mix until well combined; the dough should be soft but thick, like a thick caramel. Fold in the macadamias.

3. It's best to bake these one batch of six at a time because they are a bit precious. They bake quickly, though, so don't worry about it taking too long. Drop 6 tablespoons of batter onto the parchment paper about 3 inches apart; the cookies will spread. Err on the side of

Macadamia Lace Cookies

caution with tablespoon size; try not to go too big. Let batter sit for about a minute so that it spreads and settles just a bit before baking.

4. Bake for 6 minutes, keeping a close eye so the cookies do not burn. Remove the cookies from the oven and let them cool on the sheets for 5 minutes. They will be very soft when you take them out of the oven, but don't worry, they will firm up. You should be able to just slide the whole shebang, parchment paper and all, onto a wire rack to cool the rest of the way. Don't try to lift them from the parchment paper until they are 100 percent fully cooled, unless you want a deformed cookie. Continue with the remainder of the batter. Store in a tightly sealed container.

Morsels

If you can only find salted macadamias that is fine, just leave the salt out of the recipe.

OOH LA LAS

VEGAN OREOS, FINALLY! Oh wait, Oreos are already vegan. But still—these are even *more* vegan. All that deep black cocoa taste and creamy filling, none of those ingredients you can't pronounce. These aren't difficult, but the high volume makes them a bit of a project. Get the family together and have some fun with it! You will need a lot of parchment paper so make sure you have it before starting the recipe. For time management, make the filling while the cookies are baking.

FOR THE COOKIES:
- ¾ cup nonhydrogenated vegetable shortening, at room temperature
- 1 cup sugar
- 2 teaspoons pure vanilla extract
- ½ cup nondairy milk
- 1½ cups all-purpose flour
- ½ cup Dutch cocoa powder
- ¼ cup black cocoa powder
- 2 teaspoons cornstarch
- ½ teaspoon salt
- ¼ teaspoon baking soda

FOR THE FILLING:
- ¼ cup nonhydrogenated margarine, softened
- ¼ cup nonhydrogenated vegetable shortening, at room temperature
- 2½ to 3 cups powdered sugar
- 1 teaspoon pure vanilla extract

1. In a mixing bowl, cream the shortening and sugar with a hand mixer on medium speed. When light and fluffy (about a minute) add the vanilla and nondairy milk and mix. Add the remaining ingredients and mix until the dough holds together.
2. If it's fairly cold in your kitchen, there is no need to chill the dough. If it's a particularly hot day or your kitchen is very warm, chill the dough for 10 minutes or so.
3. Preheat oven to 325°F. Divide the dough into four pieces and roll

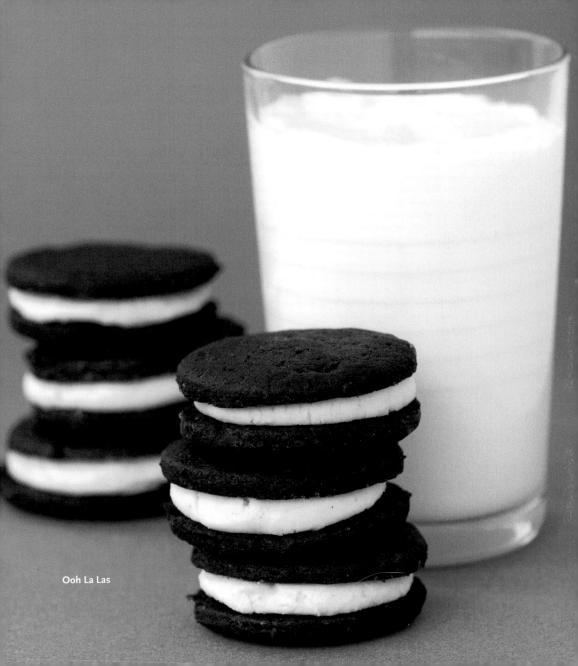

Ooh La Las

each into a ball. Place a piece of parchment paper on a flat surface. Flatten a ball of dough onto the parchment, and place another piece of parchment over it to keep the dough from sticking. Roll the dough out into a circle that is roughly 10 inches in circumference. It should be about ⅛ inch thick. Now use a 1½-inch cookie cutter to make circles in the dough. Leave about ¾-inch of space between each circle. Now lift the remaining dough away from the circles. If the dough isn't lifting easily, transfer to the fridge for 5 minutes or so.

4. Now transfer the entire piece of parchment onto the cookie sheet. No need to move the dough with a spatula, lest it get crushed. Just move the whole shebang. If your cookie sheets are big enough, you should be able to fit two rounds of dough on one sheet, although you may have to trim the parchment paper.

5. Bake for 12 minutes, then let cookies cool on the baking sheet for 5 minutes. Transfer them to wire racks to cool completely. Repeat the process with the remaining dough, and roll the scraps together, flatten and cut out more cookies until all the dough is used up.

PREPARE THE FILLING:

1. Use a hand mixer on medium-high speed to cream together the margarine and shortening. Add the powdered sugar in about ½-cup increments until thoroughly combined. It should be stiff and pliable. Mix in the vanilla. Refrigerate the filling until ready to use.

TO ASSEMBLE:

1. Roll the filling into grape-size (but round) pieces. Smoosh each piece into the flat side of a cookie. Sandwich another cookie onto the top of that and gently push down until the filling is relatively flush with the edges. Store in a tightly sealed container. If it's hot in your kitchen, refrigerate until ready to eat.

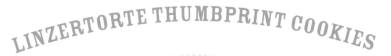

LINZERTORTE THUMBPRINT COOKIES

MAKES 20 COOKIES

EVERYONE'S FAVORITE AUSTRIAN HAZELNUT RASPBERRY COOKIE has gone thumbprint. A seriously hazelnutty cookie dough is rolled in chopped hazelnuts and filled with raspberry jam. We know hazelnut butter is super expensive, so if you would like to use almond butter instead then go for it, just expect less of an intense hazelnut taste.

⅓ cup canola oil
½ cup packed brown sugar
½ cup hazelnut butter
⅓ cup nondairy milk
1 teaspoon pure vanilla extract
1½ cups all-purpose flour
2 tablespoons cornstarch
½ teaspoon salt
¼ teaspoon baking powder
½ cup hazelnuts, finely chopped
About ⅓ cup raspberry jam

1. In a large mixing bowl, use a fork to vigorously mix the oil, sugar, and hazelnut butter. Mix in the nondairy milk and vanilla. Sift in the flour, cornstarch, salt, and baking powder and mix well until a stiff dough forms.

2. Preheat oven to 350 F. Line two baking sheets with parchment paper. Have a small bowl of water handy. Spread the chopped nuts onto a dinner plate.

3. Roll the dough into a walnut-size ball. Dip very briefly in water and firmly roll in the hazelnuts until coated. Place on a baking sheet and use either the non-spoon side of a wooden spoon or your thumb to make a deep indent in the cookie. Use your free hand to hold the cookie in place and make sure it keeps its shape. You should be able to fit all twenty cookies onto one baking sheet; they don't spread.

Linzertorte Thumbprint Cookies

4. Spoon about a teaspoon of raspberry jam into each cookie. A baby spoon works great for this! Bake for about 18 minutes. Remove the cookies from the oven and let them cool on the baking sheets for 5 minutes. Transfer them to a wire rack to cool completely. Store in a tightly sealed container.

Morsels

The easiest way to chop the hazelnuts is in a food processor fit with a metal blade. The texture will range from mealy to gravel size, and that's fine! Just make sure that nothing is bigger than a pea or you'll run into trouble when you're rolling the dough in the nuts.

SLICED AND ROLLED COOKIES

BUTTERY SHORTBREADS, **CRUNCHY BISCOTTI,** and toothsome graham crackers—no café would be complete without them and neither is your cookie jar. It may seem like these types of treats take a lot more effort, but it's really a give and take. Yes, you need to have a bit of precision when you slice them, but they're also less time consuming because you aren't forming a bunch of individual cookies. This chapter also has some of our favorite ingredients lists; green tea, chai, grapefruit— you're sure to find a fun new favorite flavor to dunk into your vintage tea cups.

CHOCOLATE CHIP CHAI SPICE SHORTBREAD

MAKES ABOUT 2-1/2 DOZEN COOKIES

You can sip chai tea while eating chocolate, or eat chai spiced-chocolate, or just nibble on buttery-tasting shortbread. It could also be annoying to have to eat and drink all three of those things at the same time. So we give you a crisp, richly flavored shortbread finger filled with both warming chai spices *and* bits of dark chocolate. Problem solved. The addition of actual chai tea is optional but there if you need maximum chai goodness.

½ cup nonhydrogenated vegetable shortening
½ cup nonhydrogenated margarine, slightly softened
¾ cup powdered sugar, sifted
½ teaspoon pure vanilla extract
1 cup all-purpose flour
1 cup whole wheat pastry flour
1½ teaspoons ground cinnamon
1 teaspoon ground cardamom
¼ teaspoon ground cloves
¼ teaspoon ground nutmeg
A generous pinch each ground coriander and ground black pepper
¼ teaspoon baking soda
¼ teaspoon salt
1 teaspoon chai tea leaf blend, about the contents of 1 tea bag

4 ounces dark chocolate, finely chopped or generous ½ cup chocolate chips

1. Preheat oven to 350°F. Line two baking sheets with parchment paper.
2. Using electric beaters in a large bowl, cream together the shortening and margarine till smooth. Fold in the powdered sugar and vanilla, then cream again with beaters till smooth and creamy.
3. In a separate bowl, sift together the all-purpose flour, whole wheat pastry flour, cinnamon, cardamom, cloves, nutmeg, coriander, pepper,

baking soda, salt, and optional chai tea. Fold half this mixture into the creamed shortening mixture to moisten all ingredients. Fold in the remaining flour mixture till a dense dough forms. Fold in the chocolate; knead the dough three or four times to completely incorporate the chocolate.

4. Divide the dough and form two logs approximately 8 x 3 inches and about ½ inch thick. With a thin, sharp knife carefully slice logs into ½-inch-thick slices. Use a spatula to carefully transfer the slices to baking sheets, placing each slice about 2 inches apart. If a slice crumbles during slicing or transfer, simply press any crumbling bits into the cookie slice when it's on the sheet.

5. Bake shortbread for 12 to 14 minutes till slightly puffed yet firm and the edges are just turning golden. Allow the cookies to cool for 5 minutes on the baking sheets before using a spatula to transfer them to wire racks.

✳ *Morsels* ✳

✦ You may encounter some frustrating crumbliness when slicing this dough while attempting to slice through chunky chocolate chips. A better solution is to use finely chopped dark chocolate instead of chips. Use a heavy knife to chop by hand either a chocolate bar or chocolate chips to create fine bits of chocolate.

✦ If the dough is very soft and difficult to work with, try chilling it after forming logs. Chill for 30 minutes before slicing.

Chocolate Chip Chai Spice Shortbread

Coffeehouse Hermits

COFFEEHOUSE HERMITS

MAKES 16 LARGE COOKIES

HAVE YOU SEEN HERMITS RESIDING IN COFFEEHOUSES? As in the cozy molasses spice cookie, that is. Soft and spicy in the center and crunchy on the edges, these raisin-y slice cookies get an extra grown-up jolt with brewed coffee, which also helps gives them rich, deep color. Gobble them up with a steaming cup of orange spice tea, cocoa, or even coffee, just in case you do indeed live in a coffeehouse.

½ cup canola oil
½ cup strong, thick black coffee, cooled to room temp
⅓ cup molasses
⅔ cup sugar, plus additional for sprinkling
2¼ cups all-purpose flour
1 teaspoon baking powder
½ teaspoon baking soda
1 teaspoon ground cinnamon
½ teaspoon ground cloves
½ teaspoon ground ginger
A generous pinch finely ground black pepper
½ teaspoon salt
1 generous cup dark raisins

1. In a large bowl, whisk together the oil, coffee, molasses, and sugar until thick. Sift in the flour, baking powder, baking soda, cinnamon, cloves, ginger, black pepper, and salt. Fold in the dry ingredients till almost completely moistened, then fold in the raisins till a soft dough forms.

2. Chill the dough in the refrigerator (no need to remove from the bowl) for 30 minutes. In the meantime, preheat the oven to 350°F. Line two baking sheets with parchment paper.

3. After dough is chilled, lightly moisten your hands and divide the dough in half. Form it into two logs on top of parchment paper, each

measuring about 13 inches long and 3½ inches wide. Leave 3 to 4 inches of room between logs as the dough will spread when baking. Sprinkle the tops of logs with additional sugar and gently press into dough.

4. Bake 24 to 26 minutes until the edges are lightly browned and the logs feel slightly firm. Cracked tops are fine, even traditionally desired with this cookie. Allow the logs to cool for 15 minutes, then with scissors or a sharp knife slice the parchment paper between the logs in two. Gently slide each log with its parchment paper onto a cutting board. With a sharp knife, slice the logs into 2-inch-wide slices, using a single downward motion with the knife. Carefully move each slice onto wire racks to complete cooling.

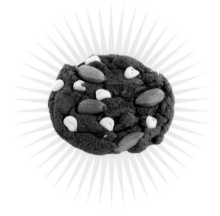

CHOCOLATE CHIP MINT LEAF ICEBOX COOKIES

MAKES ABOUT 2 DOZEN COOKIES

THIS IS A TRUE STORY FROM TERRY: "As a kid I thought that adding a handful of dry mint leaves from the garden to chocolate chip cookie batter would create the best flavor combo ever, mint chocolate chip. I hadn't quite grasped the concept of flavor extracts yet. The resulting cookies were edible if not just a little twiggy, but not as minty as one would hope. Since then I've learned just a little bit about baking extracts. But I still put green things in cookies."

Here's a sophisticated version of this cookie straight outta childhood. Tiny, bright-green flecks of fresh mint give these buttery cookies a unique appearance and herbal finish. And a little mint extract comes in strong for that necessary cool minty aftertaste.

½ cup fresh mint leaves, lightly packed
½ cup nonhydrogenated margarine, softened
½ cup nonhydrogenated vegetable shortening
1 cup plus 2 tablespoons sugar
1½ teaspoons pure vanilla extract
1 teaspoon mint extract
¼ cup nondairy milk
1⅔ cups all-purpose flour
⅓ cup cornstarch
¼ teaspoon salt
½ teaspoon baking soda
1 cup chocolate chips (lightly chop chips if they are very large; this will make slicing the dough much easier)

1. Wash the mint leaves and pat them dry with a towel or spin them in a salad spinner. Remove any stems and with a heavy knife mince the leaves very fine.

2. In a large bowl, using an electric hand mixer, cream together the margarine, shortening, and sugar until light and fluffy, about 3 minutes. Scrape down the sides of the bowl often. Beat in the vanilla and mint extracts. Add nondairy milk and beat until creamy. Sift in the flour, cornstarch, salt, and baking

soda and mix to form a soft dough. Using a rubber spatula, fold in the finely chopped mint and chocolate chips. Dough will be slightly sticky.

3. Scrape the dough, with a rubber spatula, onto a large sheet of wax paper. Form a log about 2 inches wide and 12 inches long, taking hold of the ends of the wax paper and gently tugging to create a rounder log of dough. Wrap and tuck in the ends of the wax paper and chill the dough till very firm, at least 2 hours or overnight.

4. Preheat oven to 350°F. Line two baking sheets with parchment paper. Slice the dough into ½-inch-thick slices, place them at least 2 inches apart on the sheets (cookies will spread), and bake 12 to 14 minutes till the edges start to brown. Remove the cookies from the oven and allow them to cool 5 minutes before carefully lifting them with a spatula onto wire racks to cool. Store in a loosely covered container.

Morsels

For best results really chop that mint very fine, as fine as you possibly can. Tiny specks of green leaves look cuter than large ones.

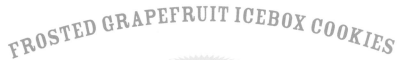

FROSTED GRAPEFRUIT ICEBOX COOKIES

MAKES ABOUT 2 DOZEN COOKIES

NO LONGER THE RED-FRUITED STEPCHILD, grapefruit shines front and center in these buttery square treats. You should be able to get enough zest and juice from one grapefruit, but pick up two just in case.

½ cup nonhydrogenated margarine
¼ cup nonhydrogenated vegetable shortening
½ cup sugar
1 teaspoon pure vanilla extract
¼ cup fresh red grapefruit juice
1 tablespoon red grapefruit zest
1¾ cups all-purpose flour
1 tablespoon cornstarch
½ teaspoon baking powder
¼ teaspoon salt

FOR THE GLAZE:
2 cups powdered sugar
3 to 4 tablespoons red grapefruit juice
½ teaspoon pure vanilla extract
2 tablespoons red grapefruit zest for sprinkling

1. In a large mixing bowl, with a hand mixer on medium speed, cream together the margarine and shortening. Beat in the sugar until light and fluffy. Mix in the vanilla, grapefruit juice, and grapefruit zest. Add flour, cornstarch, baking powder, and salt and beat until a soft dough forms.

2. On a piece of parchment paper form the dough into a log about 14 inches long. Roll the log up in parchment paper and rotate it, pressing the dough to square off the sides. Refrigerate for at least 2 hours and up to overnight.

3. Preheat oven to 350°F and line two baking sheets with parchment paper.

4. Remove the dough from the fridge and cut the rectangle into slices

Frosted Grapefruit Icebox Cookies

just under ½ inch thick; place them on the cookie sheets. The end slices are going to be a little wacky; that's okay, just discard them or make two weird-looking cookies.

5. Bake the cookies for 15 minutes; the edges should be lightly browned. Let the cookies cool on sheets for 5 minutes, then transfer them to a wire rack to cool completely before glazing.

MAKE THE GLAZE AND ASSEMBLE:

1. In a small mixing bowl, use a fork to mix together the sugar, grape- fruit juice, and vanilla. The glaze should fall from the fork in thick ribbons; if it seems too thin, add a little extra sugar. If too thick, add more grapefruit juice by the tea- spoon. Spoon the glaze onto the cooled cookies and spread it a bit. Sprinkle the cookies with a little grapefruit zest. Let the cookies set for at least half an hour. If it's warm in the kitchen, place them in the fridge to set. Store in a container until ready to use.

CORNMEAL POPPY SEED BISCOTTI

MAKES 18 BISCOTTI

WITH WHOLESOME CORNMEAL AND POPPY SEEDS, these golden biscotti are particularly suitable for breakfast or a light brunch. Pleasantly grainy, think of them as the crunchy (and best) part of a muffin top. A touch of lemon makes them the perfect companion to a cuppa Earl Grey.

¼ cup soy milk
2 tablespoons lemon juice
2 tablespoons ground flax seeds
½ cup canola oil
¾ cup sugar
Grated zest of 1 lemon
½ teaspoon pure vanilla extract
1⅓ cups all-purpose flour
½ cup yellow cornmeal
2 tablespoons cornstarch
1 teaspoon baking powder
½ teaspoon baking soda
½ teaspoon salt
2 tablespoons poppy seeds

1. Preheat oven to 350°F. Line a baking sheet with parchment paper.
2. In a large bowl, stir together the soy milk and lemon juice till the soy milk curdles. Beat in the flax seeds, oil, sugar, lemon zest, and vanilla till smooth.
3. Sift in the flour, cornmeal, cornstarch, baking powder, baking soda, and salt. If any large particles of cornmeal remain in the sifter, dump those into the bowl also. Add the poppy seeds. Stir to form a soft dough.
4. Form a log about 10 to 11 inches long by 4 inches wide, using a rubber spatula to even edges and flatten the end sides of the log. Bake for 28 to 30 minutes until the log is puffed and firm. Some cracking is okay. Place the baking sheet on a wire rack, turn off the oven, and allow the log to cool for at least 45

minutes. If any edges of the log are too browned, gently trim them off with a sharp, heavy knife.

5. Preheat oven again, to 325°F. Very carefully slide the log off the baking sheet onto a cutting board. With a sharp, heavy knife, cut the log into ½-inch-thick slices, using one quick and firm motion, pressing down into the log. Very gently, move the slices to the baking sheet (sliding a chef's knife underneath works well), standing them on their bottom edge if possible.

6. Rebake the slices for 26 to 28 minutes. The slices should appear dry, but do not allow them to get too browned. Allow the biscotti to cool 10 minutes on the baking sheet, then carefully move them to wire racks to complete cooling (warm biscotti may be fragile). Store in a loosely covered container.

Morsels

If the biscotti seem to crumble when the from-above slicing method is used, try placing your chef's knife on one side of the cookie log and rocking the knife blade in one firm motion to the other side.

Gingerbread Biscotti

GINGERBREAD BISCOTTI

FOR THE NEVER-CAN-GET-ENOUGH-BISCOTTI-AND-CANDIED-GINGER people in your life. Candied ginger and molasses make 'em chewy in the center, and the traditional double baking gives them that necessary biscotti crunch on the edges. These are lovely served naked or sussed up for the holidays with a drizzle of LEMON GLAZE (page 38) or melted white vegan chocolate.

¼ cup molasses
⅔ cup sugar
2 tablespoons ground flax seeds
½ cup canola oil
2 tablespoons nondairy milk
1 teaspoon pure vanilla extract
1¾ cups all-purpose flour
2 teaspoons ground ginger
1½ teaspoons ground cinnamon
½ teaspoon ground nutmeg
1½ teaspoons baking powder
½ teaspoon salt
4 ounces candied ginger, finely chopped

1. Preheat oven to 350°F. Line a baking sheet with parchment paper.
2. In a large bowl, beat together molasses, sugar, flax seeds, oil, nondairy milk, and vanilla with a wire whisk until smooth.
3. Sift in the flour, ground ginger, cinnamon, nutmeg, baking powder, and salt. Stir with a wooden spoon or rubber spatula to form a smooth dough, then knead in the chopped candied ginger, pushing any bits that pop out back into the dough.
4. Form a log about 11 inches long by 4 inches wide, using a rubber spatula to even the edges and flatten the end sides of the log. Bake for 28 to 30 minutes until the log is puffed and firm but not too brown. It will spread a little, and some cracking is okay. Place the baking sheet on a

wire rack, turn off the oven, and allow the log to cool for at least 45 minutes. If any edges of the log are too browned, gently trim them off with a sharp, heavy knife.

5. Preheat oven to 325°F. Very carefully, slide the log off the baking sheet and onto a cutting board. With a sharp, heavy knife, cut log into ½-inch-thick slices, using one quick and firm motion, pressing down into the log. Very gently move slices to the baking sheet, standing them on their bottom edge if possible. Rebake the slices for 22 to 24 minutes. The slices should appear dry and slightly toasted, but do not allow them to get too browned. Allow the biscotti to cool 10 minutes on the baking sheet, then carefully move them to wire racks to complete cooling (warm biscotti may be fragile). Store in a loosely covered container.

Morsels

Substitute ¾ cup whole wheat pastry flour for all-purpose flour to add a little whole-grain stuff to these cookies.

GREEN TEA WALNUT BISCOTTI

MAKES 18 BISCOTTI

FANS OF ALL THINGS GREEN will love this nutty biscotti the color of envy, money, or in this case, actual tea. The grassy-bitter matcha green tea plus deeply toasted walnuts equals a nuanced blend of sophisticated flavors. Make these biscotti with a little whole-grain pastry flour and you have a healthful treat to serve up alongside guess what, more green tea!

¼ cup nondairy milk
4 teaspoons matcha green tea powder
2 tablespoons ground flax seeds
½ cup canola oil
¾ cup sugar
1 teaspoon pure vanilla extract
1 cup all-purpose flour
½ cup whole wheat pastry flour
2 tablespoons cornstarch
1 teaspoon baking powder
¼ teaspoon salt
4 ounces walnut halves (about 1¼ cups)

1. Preheat oven to 350°F. Line a baking sheet with parchment paper.
2. Pour the nondairy milk into a large bowl and add the green tea powder. Use a wire whisk to beat until no lumps remain. Beat in flax seeds until smooth. Add oil, sugar, and vanilla and mix to combine.
3. Sift in the flours, cornstarch, baking powder, and salt. Stir to form a smooth dough, then knead in the walnut halves, pushing any nuts that pop out back into the dough.
4. Form a log about 10 inches long by 4 inches, using a rubber spatula to even edges and flatten end sides of log. Bake for 30 minutes until the log is puffed and firm. Some cracking is okay. Place the baking sheet on a wire rack, turn off the oven, and allow the log to cool for at least 45 minutes. If any edges of the log are too browned, gently trim them off with a sharp, heavy knife.

5. Preheat oven to 325°F. Very carefully, slide the log off the baking sheet and onto a cutting board. With a sharp, heavy knife slice log into ½-inch thick slices, using one quick and firm motion, pressing down into the log. Very gently move the slices to a baking sheet, standing them on their bottom edge if possible. Rebake the slices for 26 to 28 minutes. The biscotti should appear dry and nuts should be lightly toasted. Allow the biscotti to cool 10 minutes on the baking sheet, then carefully move them to wire racks to complete cooling (warm biscotti may be fragile). Store in a loosely covered container.

Variation

PISTACHIO GREEN TEA BISCOTTI: The ultimate naturally green cookie. Omit the walnuts and substitute 4 ounces of green, unsalted, and unshelled pistachio nuts.

Morsels

The dark green dough will turn a lighter shade after baking. Some varieties of matcha powder may have an intense hue that remains bright green through the whole baking process. We don't have a specific brand to recommend, but if you should be so lucky to score some you could have biscotti so amazingly green it'll make a frog blush. Use pure powdered matcha green tea without added sugar. Definitely no green tea–flavored beverage mixes either.

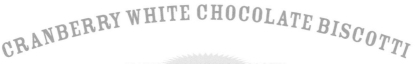

CRANBERRY WHITE CHOCOLATE BISCOTTI

MAKES AROUND 16 BISCOTTI

A FRUITY BISCOTTI WITH TART CRANBERRIES, sweet white chocolate chips, a dash of orange, and a hint of allspice. This is perfect for the winter holidays or with some Lady Grey tea. If you don't have vegan white chocolate chips (page 16), don't use regular chocolate chips because they would be overwhelming. Instead use macadamia nuts since they're nice and creamy (for a nut).

⅓ cup almond milk
2 tablespoons ground flax seeds
2 teaspoons orange zest
¾ cup sugar
½ cup canola oil
1 teaspoon pure vanilla extract
1⅔ cups all-purpose flour
2 tablespoons arrowroot powder
2 teaspoons baking powder
¼ teaspoon allspice
½ teaspoon salt
½ cup white chocolate chips
½ cup dried cranberries

1. Preheat oven to 350°F. Line a baking sheet with parchment paper.
2. In a large mixing bowl, whisk together the almond milk and flax seeds, beating for about 30 seconds.

Mix in the orange zest, sugar, oil, and vanilla. Sift in the flour, arrowroot powder, baking powder, allspice, and salt. Stir to combine, and just before the dough comes together knead in the chocolate chips and cranberries. Knead to form a stiff dough. If cranberries and chips pop out just press them back in as well as you can.

3. On the parchment, form the dough into a log and press it into a rectangle about 12 inches long and 4 inches wide. Bake for 26 to 28 minutes till lightly puffed and browned. Let the log cool on the baking sheet for about 30 minutes.

4. Preheat oven to 325°F. Carefully transfer the baked log to a cutting board. With a heavy, very sharp knife, cut ½-inch-thick slices. The best way to do this is in one motion, pushing down; don't "saw" the slices off or they could crumble. Stand slices, curved sides up, ½ inch apart on baking sheet, and bake for 20 to 25 minutes, until biscotti appear dry and toasted. Transfer the biscotti to a wire rack to cool completely.

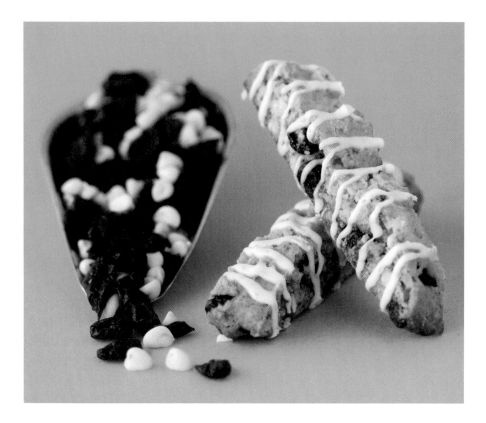

KEY LIME SHORTBREAD ROUNDS

MAKES A LITTLE OVER 2 DOZEN COOKIES

NO TIME OR CASH FOR A TRIP TO THE FLORIDA KEYS? Here's an honest icebox cookie that packs fresh tropical lime flavor. Its pleasantly crunchy, sugared edge doesn't require SPF 30, or swimsuit shopping, or sand in your shoes. Plus the only heat you'll have to deal with is turning on the oven and ... okay, all right, we know it's no substitute for a vacation, but at least these rich little shortbread rounds are pretty to look at and simple to throw together.

½ cup nonhydrogenated vegetable shortening

⅓ cup nonhydrogenated margarine, softened

1 cup plus 2 tablespoons powdered sugar, sifted

¼ cup lime juice, preferably concentrated Key lime juice

½ teaspoon pure vanilla extract

2 generous teaspoons finely grated lime zest (about 2 small limes, 4 to 5 Key limes)

2 cups all-purpose flour

¼ teaspoon baking soda

¼ teaspoon salt

Large crystal decorating sugar for rolling, about ¼ cup

1. In a large bowl, using electric beaters, cream together the shortening and margarine until fluffy and creamy. Scrape the bowl then beat in the powdered sugar until thick and smooth. Add the lime juice, vanilla, and lime zest and beat for about 30 seconds to mix, scraping down the sides of the bowl occasionally.

2. In a medium bowl, sift together the flour, baking soda, and salt. Add half of this mixture to the shortening mixture and beat to moisten the ingredients. Add the remaining flour mixture and beat for about

1 minute until a soft ball of dough forms.

3. Divide the dough in half and place each half on a separate large sheet of wax paper. Roll each half into a log about 7 to 8 inches long by 1½ to 1¾ inches thick in diameter. Sprinkle about 2 tablespoons of decorating sugar in a line onto wax paper and roll a log to coat the outsides in sugar. Repeat with the remaining dough log. Wrap each log tightly in wax paper and chill for at least 1 hour till very firm.

4. Preheat oven to 350°F. Line two baking sheets with parchment paper. With a thin, sharp knife, cut ½-inch slices of dough. Place slices on the cookie sheets, leaving about 2 inches of space between cookies. Bake for 10 to 12 minutes or until slightly puffed and edges are just beginning to turn golden. Do not overbake, as the cookies will rapidly turn very golden brown. Allow the cookies to cool for 5 minutes before transferring them to wire racks to complete cooling.

❋ *Morsels* ❋

✦ For the most intense lime flavor use concentrated Key lime juice. Look for it at your nearby gourmet grocery where the concentrated lemon juice is usually stocked. Of course you can also use fresh lime juice, the flavor will just be less intense. Or perhaps you lead a charmed life, and your produce aisle stocks those cute little fresh Key limes.

✦ India Tree brand makes a gorgeously green "Emerald Green" decorating sugar. But demerara sugar or untinted, large-grained sugar works just as well if you prefer a less verdant cookie.

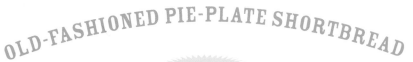

OLD-FASHIONED PIE-PLATE SHORTBREAD

MAKES 12 GENEROUS SHORTBREAD WEDGES

BIG WEDGES OF OLD-SCHOOL SHORTBREAD JUST SCREAM "uppity tea time" but are still so ridiculously charming that they feel right at home with the milk 'n' cookie–loving masses. Rich and sweet, but not overly so, this shortbread is fantastic flavored with rose water or lavender flowers for something different or with just pure vanilla extract.

Baking these requires little craftiness on your part. Just press the dough into a standard shallow tart (quiche-type) pan, bake, and you're suddenly a fabulous tea-party hostess/host.

1 cup nonhydrogenated margarine, slightly softened, plus more for greasing
⅔ cup sugar
2½ teaspoons pure vanilla extract
2 cups all-purpose flour
⅓ cup cornstarch
1 additional teaspoon sugar, for sprinkling

1. Preheat oven to 350°F. Lightly grease a 10-inch shallow tart pan, the metal kind with a fluted edge and removable bottom.

2. In a large bowl, beat the margarine and sugar together with an electric beater or even a standing electric mixer. Scrape the sides of the bowl frequently with a rubber spatula and beat the mixture till very light and creamy, about 5 minutes. Stir in the vanilla.

3. Sift together the flour and cornstarch. Add half this mixture to the beaten margarine mixture, using the rubber spatula to fold in the flour first so that it doesn't fly all over the place when using the mixer beaters. Beat until mostly combined, then add the rest of the flour mixture using the spatula as

before. Continue to stir until all the flour and cornstarch are absorbed and dough is crumbly yet soft and moist.

4. Pour the crumbly dough into the prepared tart pan and distribute evenly. Using your fingers, firmly press the dough down into the pan so that the crumbles smoosh together; if it feels a little like you're making pie crust, in a way you certainly are! Make sure to also press the dough into the fluted edges of the pan; try using the curved tip of a butter knife. Press down everything as evenly and firmly as possible.

5. Use a fork to gently poke into the dough at even intervals, sinking fork tines about halfway through the dough. Place the tart pan on a baking sheet in the center of the oven rack and bake 30 to 32 minutes until the shortbread is slightly puffed and the edges are starting to turn pale gold. Remove the pan from the oven and set it on a wooden cutting board. Sprinkle the shortbread with 1 teaspoon of sugar. Let cool for 15 minutes.

6. Use a thin, sharp knife to slice the warm shortbread into twelve wedges. Place the entire pan on a wire rack and allow it to cool at least another 30 minutes before removing the wedges from the pan and serving. Store completely cooled shortbread in a tightly covered container.

Morsels

Regular granulated sugar gives this shortbread a classic, slightly crunchy texture. If you prefer a more delicate shortbread try using caster (superfine) sugar instead.

VEGAN COOKIES INVADE YOUR COOKIE JAR

Variations

ROSE WATER SHORTBREAD: Reduce the vanilla to 1 teaspoon and add 1½ teaspoons rose water.

LAVENDER SHORTBREAD: A beautiful and thrilling shortbread with the intense floral aroma and citrusy, slightly anise-like flavor of lavender. Reduce the vanilla to ½ teaspoon and add 2 tablespoons organic (or look for unsprayed, food-grade) dried lavender flowers to the dough along with the remainder of the flour.

EARL GREY SHORTBREAD: Same as lavender, but instead use 2 tablespoons of loose-leaf Earl Grey tea.

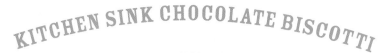

KITCHEN SINK CHOCOLATE BISCOTTI

MAKES 18 BISCOTTI

AS YOU PROBABLY GUESSED WE'RE BIG-TIME BISCOTTI FANS HERE. What's not to love about basically baking up one huge cookie, then transforming it into a bunch of crisp little ones built for dunking into tea, coffee, or almond milk? Here is our favorite all-purpose chocolate biscotti that's ideal for those times when you can't decide between chocolate chip, almonds, espresso beans, apricots … just use them all! The dough can support up to 1 generous cup of mix-ins.

¼ cup nondairy milk
2 tablespoons ground flax seeds
½ cup canola oil
1 cup sugar
2 teaspoons pure vanilla extract
1 cup all-purpose flour
½ cup whole wheat pastry flour
½ cup Dutch cocoa powder
1¼ teaspoons baking powder
¼ teaspoon salt
⅓ cup *each* of *two or three* of the following: chocolate chips, whole almonds, vegan white chocolate chips, dried cherries, raisins, vegan butterscotch chips, cacao nibs, chocolate-covered espresso beans, whole peanuts, chopped dates, freeze-dried raspberries, crushed peppermint candies, cashews, chopped dried apricots, walnuts, macadamia nuts, dried cranberries

1. Preheat oven to 350°F. Line a baking sheet with parchment paper.
2. In a large bowl, beat together the nondairy milk and flax seeds until smooth. Add oil, sugar, and vanilla and mix to combine.
3. Sift in the flour, whole wheat pastry flour, cocoa powder, baking powder, and salt. Stir to form a smooth dough, then knead in up to 1 cup of mix-ins, pushing any pieces that pop out back into the dough.

4. Form a log about 10 inches long by 4 inches wide, using a rubber spatula to even the edges and flatten the ends. Bake for 30 minutes until the log is puffed and firm. Some cracking is okay. Place the baking sheet on a wire rack, turn off the oven, and allow the log to cool for at least 45 minutes. If any edges of the log are too browned, gently trim them off with a sharp, heavy knife.

5. Preheat oven to 325°F. Very carefully, slide the log off the baking sheet and onto a cutting board. With a sharp, heavy knife cut the log into ½-inch-thick slices, using one quick and firm motion, pressing down into the log. Very gently move the slices to the baking sheet, standing them on their bottom edge if possible. Bake the slices for 26 to 28 minutes. The slices should appear dry, and any nuts used should be lightly toasted. Allow the biscotti to cool 10 minutes on the baking sheet, then carefully move them to wire racks to complete cooling (warm biscotti may be fragile). Store in a loosely covered container.

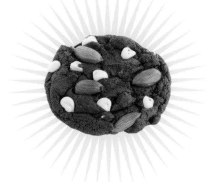

GRAHAM CRACKERS

FINALLY, A GRAHAM CRACKER THAT IS HASSLE-FREE! Most graham cracker recipes call for chilling the dough, but we want graham crackers *now*, not in three hours! These are also relatively healthy for a sweet treat, with a hearty wheaty crunch. To add to the beauty of this recipe, everything gets done with just a large mixing bowl and a fork.

1½ cups whole wheat flour
⅓ cup sugar
½ teaspoon baking soda
½ teaspoon cinnamon
A scant ½ teaspoon salt
¼ cup oil
2 tablespoons molasses
1 teaspoon pure vanilla extract
¼ cup nondairy milk

1. Preheat oven to 350°F. Line a light-colored baking sheet with parchment paper.
2. In a large bowl mix together flour, sugar, baking soda, cinnamon, and salt. Make a well in the middle and pour in oil, molasses, and vanilla. Give the liquid ingredients a quick whisk with a fork and then continue mixing until everything is well combined and crumbly.
3. Drizzle in the nondairy milk and combine. Use your hands to knead the dough a few times until it holds together; add an extra tablespoon of nondairy milk if needed. You should be able to form a pliable ball of dough.
4. Line a work surface with parchment paper. Place the dough on the parchment and work into a rectangle. Flatten it a bit with the palms of your hand and sprinkle with flour. Use a rolling pin to roll the dough into a rectangle that is

roughly 10 x 14 inches. The dough should be about ⅛ inch thick. If the edges look crumbly, that's okay.

5. Cut the edges off so that you have a relatively even 12 x 8-inch rectangle. Cut the dough into eight crackers; to do this evenly, use a sharp paring knife to slice the dough in quarters. Then cut widthwise again on either side of the center widthwise cut. That probably made it sound confusing; read it slowly.

6. Use a very thin, flexible spatula to transfer the crackers to a baking sheet. It helps if you spray the spatula with cooking spray so that it slips off the crackers easily.

7. Gather up the scraps of dough and form them into a ball, then roll it out into a 4 by 8-inch rectangle, or whatever size you can manage. We were able to get four more crackers out of the deal, but your mileage may vary. Cut the edges evenly and slice into four crackers, then transfer them to the baking sheet.

8. Score each cookie with a fork four times in two columns. You don't need to poke all the way through. Bake for 12 to 14 minutes—14 minutes will give you nice crispy crackers, 12 will be better for making ice-cream sammiches.

9. Let the crackers cool completely on the baking sheet.

Variation

CINNAMON SUGAR GRAHAM CRACKERS: Mix together 1 tablespoon sugar and ½ teaspoon cinnamon. Sprinkle the sugar mixture on top of the crackers after rolling and before scoring.

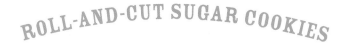

ROLL-AND-CUT SUGAR COOKIES

MAKES ABOUT 3 DOZEN COOKIES,

depending on the size of your cutters

AN ALL-PURPOSE, FUN-LOVING, BUTTERY SUGAR COOKIE meant for rollin' and cuttin' into any shape your heart desires. Including the shape of your heart if that's what you're into. Industrious types (definitely not us) will want to decorate these with tinted CONFECTIONER'S ICING **(page 224),** tiny candies, sprinkles, etc. They are also a simple pleasure to eat as-is, naked and unadorned.

Try experimenting with rolling the dough into varying degrees of thickness for varying crispness, but keep a careful eye on these cookies when baking if you're rolling them 1/8 inch or thinner.

2⅓ cups all-purpose flour
2 tablespoons cornstarch
¼ teaspoon salt
¼ teaspoon baking powder
½ cup nonhydrogenated margarine, slightly softened
½ cup nonhydrogenated vegetable shortening
1 cup sugar
2 teaspoons pure vanilla extract
½ teaspoon almond, lemon, maple, or other flavor extract
¼ cup vanilla nondairy milk

1. In a mixing bowl, sift together the flour, cornstarch, salt, and baking powder. Set aside.

2. In a large mixing bowl, use electric beaters to cream together the margarine, shortening, and sugar until light and fluffy, at least 4 minutes. Scrape the sides of the bowl occasionally with a rubber spatula. Beat in the vanilla extract, the flavor extract, and the nondairy milk to combine. Beat in half the flour mixture until moistened, then care-

fully mix in the remaining flour mixture to form a soft dough.

3. Divide the mixture in two and pat into discs about 1 inch thick. Wrap each disc in plastic wrap and chill for several hours or overnight.

4. Preheat oven to 350°F. Line two baking sheets with parchment paper. Lightly flour a large, clean work surface. Roll the dough to a ⅜-inch thickness and cut into shapes with cookie cutters. If the dough seems too stiff to roll or cracks too much, let it rest at room temperature for 10 minutes, then try rolling again. Pull away excess dough and use a thin metal spatula to carefully lift cookies onto cookie sheets, leaving an inch of space between cookies. Bake for 8 to 10 minutes or until the cookies have just started to turn golden around the edges. Remove the cookies from the oven and let them cool on sheets for 5 minutes before using that spatula again to transfer them to wire racks. Use only completely cooled cookies for decorating or filling. Store in a tightly covered container for softer cookies; store loosely covered for crisper cookies.

Variation

CINNAMON SAND TARTS: Thin, crispy, and just the right touch of spice. When you want shaped sugar cookies with that little something extra.

Roll dough very thin, ⅛ inch or slightly thinner. Cut into shapes, brush with a little soy creamer or nondairy milk, and sprinkle with cinnamon sugar (3 tablespoons sugar plus ½ teaspoon ground cinnamon). Bake as directed for 6 to 7 minutes until the edges are golden, watching carefully so cookies don't get too brown. Cool the same as regular sugar cut-outs.

✳ *Morsels* ✳

- ✦ Cookie dough gets a little tougher and drier each time you reroll it, so for best results don't reroll more than once. Wrap dough scraps in plastic wrap and chill in the refrigerator between rolling out and cutting cookies.
- ✦ Make a quick and cheap BIG rolling space by using masking tape to secure the edges of a nice big piece of wax paper onto a stable rolling surface.

★ ★ ★

CONFECTIONER'S ICING

Easy icing that dries to a hard, matte finish. If desired, divide this recipe into separate portions in small mixing bowls and tint each one a different color, evenly blending in food coloring with a fork or whisk.

> 4 cups sifted powdered sugar
> 4 tablespoons nondairy milk
> ½ teaspoon pure vanilla extract

1. In a large mixing bowl, whisk together all the ingredients using a fork or a wire whisk until smooth. Combine to form a glaze that can be easily spread with an icing spatula or piped from a pastry bag with a very small round tip.
2. If the icing is too thick, whisk in 1 teaspoon at a time of either nondairy milk or water. If too thin, whisk in more powdered sugar by the tablespoon until a desired consistency is reached.

CHOCOLATE CUT-OUT COOKIES

MAKES 3 DOZEN 2-INCH COOKIES

SO YOU'VE GOT THOSE ADORABLE COOKIE CUTTERS NOW and you've had it up to here with vanilla butter cookies. Well, good news, now fun shapes come in chocolate, too!

⅔ cup sugar
¼ cup oil
¼ cup nondairy milk
1 teaspoon pure vanilla extract
¼ teaspoon almond extract
1 cup all-purpose flour
½ cup Dutch cocoa powder
1 tablespoon cornstarch
½ teaspoon baking powder
¼ teaspoon salt

1. In a mixing bowl, vigorously mix the sugar, oil, and nondairy milk. Mix in vanilla and almond extracts.
2. Sift in the flour, cocoa powder, cornstarch, baking powder, and salt. Mix until well combined. The dough should be stiff but pliable. Divide in half, and form into discs; flatten and refrigerate for about an hour.
3. Preheat oven to 350°F. Line two baking sheets with parchment paper. Roll dough out about ⅛ inch thick onto a lightly floured surface. Use a cookie cutter to cut out shapes and a thin spatula to transfer the cookies to the baking sheets. Roll the dough scraps out to get a few more cookies.
4. Bake for 7 minutes. Let cookies cool on the baking sheets for 2 minutes before moving them to wire racks to cool completely. Store in a tightly sealed container.

GINGERBREAD CUT-OUT COOKIES

MAKES ABOUT 16 COOKIES

(depending on the size of your cutters)

WHETHER YOU'RE GOING ALL-OUT WITH YOUR DECORATING or you're a part of the gingerbread minimalist movement, this recipe is a surefire winner that will have you singing Christmas carols under your breath and then looking around to make sure no one heard you.

⅓ cup canola oil
¾ cup sugar
¼ cup molasses
¼ cup plain soy milk
2 cups whole wheat pastry flour or all-purpose flour (or a mix of both)
½ teaspoon baking soda
½ teaspoon baking powder
½ teaspoon salt

FOR THE SPICE BLEND:
½ teaspoon each ground nutmeg, cloves, and cinnamon
1½ teaspoons ground ginger

1. In a large bowl, whisk together the oil and sugar for about 3 minutes. Add the molasses and soy milk. The molasses and soy milk won't really blend with the oil but that's okay.

2. Sift in all the other dry ingredients, mixing about halfway through. When all of the dry ingredients are added, mix until a stiff dough is formed. Flatten the dough into a disc, wrap it in plastic wrap, and chill for an hour or up to 3 days in advance. If the dough chills longer than an hour you may want to let it sit for 10 minutes to warm up a bit before proceeding.

VEGAN COOKIES INVADE YOUR COOKIE JAR

3. Preheat oven to 350°F. Lightly grease two baking sheets or line them with parchment paper.

4. On a lightly floured surface, roll the dough out to a little less than ¼ inch thick. Cut out your shapes with your cookie cutters and use a thin spatula to gently place the cookies on the sheets. If you are using the cookies to decorate a tree or something, remember to punch a hole in their heads (!) before baking. Bake for 8 minutes.

5. Remove the cookies from the oven and let them cool for 2 minutes on the baking sheet, then move them to a wire rack. Wait until they are completely cool before icing.

NO-BAKE PECAN CHOCOLATES

THESE TASTE LIKE A CHOCOLATE CONFECTION from a heart-shaped box. The brown rice syrup and chocolate combo really melts in your mouth like caramel. These are super duper easy and soooo luxuriously delicious.

2 cups pecans, divided
½ cup brown rice syrup
A scant ¼ teaspoon salt
2 teaspoons pure vanilla extract (use bourbon vanilla extract from Trader Joe's if you've got it)
1 cup chocolate chips, melted (page 24)

1. Place 1 cup of the pecans in a food processor and process into coarse crumbs. Roughly chop the other cup.

2. In a medium mixing bowl, use a fork to mix together the brown rice syrup, salt, and vanilla. Mix in the pecan crumbs and chopped pecans. Last, mix in the melted chocolate.

3. Line a large cutting board or cookie tray with parchment paper. Have a bowl of water close at hand. Use a tablespoon to drop spoonfuls of the mixture onto the parchment. Wet your other hand and flatten each spoonful into rustic cookie shapes. The water will keep your hand from getting all sticky and stuff.

4. Place the cookies in the fridge until set, about an hour. If it's a hot day out, keep them chilled, but they should be fine left out if the weather's not too warm.

SWEDISH CHOCOLATE BALLS

MAKES ABOUT 2 DOZEN COOKIES

THESE TASTY, NO-BAKE CONFECTIONS ARE POPULAR IN SWEDEN, typically eaten as a snack while taking a coffee break. Easy to make and creamy, they taste like a cross between an oatmeal cookie and a chocolate truffle. And oh, look, they're wheat-free without even trying. Flaked sweetened coconut and Swedish pearl sugar (a large-grain, snow-white sugar with a crunchy texture) are traditionally used to coat these cookie balls, but do try finely chopped nuts or cookie crumbs or even crushed sweetened cereal for fun.

This adaptation of *chokladboll* is based on our friend Peter's family recipe. So we guess it's okay to call these Peter's Chocolaty Balls. There, it has been said.

3¼ cups of quick-cooking oats
A pinch of salt
1 cup plus 2 tablespoons powdered
  sugar
⅓ cup natural or Dutch cocoa powder
½ cup nonhydrogenated margarine,
  softened
½ cup chocolate or vanilla nondairy milk
  or chilled brewed coffee
1¼ teaspoons pure vanilla extract

FOR THE COATING:
1½ cups or more flaked coconut or
  finely chopped nuts or cookie
  crumbs or crushed sweetened cereal
  or 1 cup pearl sugar.

1. In a large bowl, combine the oats and salt, then sift in the powdered sugar and cocoa powder. Add the margarine and use a pastry cutter or a large fork to combine with dry ingredients, mashing to form a crumbly mixture. Pour in the nondairy milk and vanilla, stirring with a rubber spatula to form a thick, sticky dough.

2. Spread out the coconut on a large plate. If using other coatings for the cookies, spread these out into separate plates. For each cookie

scoop a generous tablespoon of dough, drop directly into the coating, roll to cover completely, and then briefly roll between your palms to form a smooth ball. Repeat with the remaining dough. If desired, chill the cookie balls for at least 30 minutes prior to serving to allow flavors and textures to meld a bit. Store in a tightly covered container in the refrigerator until ready to serve.

✺ *Morsels* ✺

◆ For a smoother texture, try whirling the oats in a blender for a few seconds. Take care not to overblend oats to a fine flour, though.

◆ Look for pearl sugar in gourmet baking supply stores or stores that sell Swedish stuff.

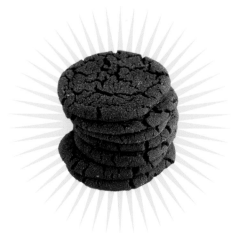

COOKIE DOUGH SCOOPS

EVERYONE KNOWS THAT UNCOOKED COOKIE DOUGH is the most all-American snack there ever was or will be. Never mind the peanuts or popcorn. Any dough in this book could be consumed straight out of the bowl, but this recipe is a classic—creamy, buttery-tasty brown sugar dough plus a generous portion of chocolate chips. And no baking soda or powder ensures no bitter aftertaste. You can enjoy these cute frozen scoops as is or roll them into a tube, store in the fridge, and slice off rounds as needed. Or fancy them up with a partial dip in melted chocolate if they don't get gobbled up immediately.

1 cup dark brown sugar
2 tablespoons sugar
¼ cup nondairy milk
½ cup nonhydrogenated margarine, softened
1½ teaspoons pure vanilla extract
1¾ cups all-purpose flour
¼ teaspoon salt
1¼ cups chocolate chips

1. In a large mixing bowl, use electric beaters to combine the sugars and the nondairy milk until the sugars are moistened. Beat in the margarine and vanilla, creaming the mixture until combined. Add the flour and salt and beat to form a soft, fluffy dough. Use a rubber spatula to fold in the chocolate chips.

2. Place a sheet of waxed paper onto a small baking sheet or cutting board that will fit into your freezer. Use a small ice cream scoop to scoop out balls of dough onto waxed paper. Freeze for 1 hour or until firm. If desired, let the cookies stand for 10 minutes to soften slightly before serving. Store cookies loosely covered in the freezer.

Variations

COOKIE DOUGH DIPPED SCOOPS: Melt 1 cup of chocolate chips (page 24) and dip the bottoms of the frozen cookies into the chocolate. Place them back on the waxed paper and freeze for 10 minutes or until the chocolate is firm.

GLUTEN-FREE COOKIE SCOOPS: Since there's no baking required it's easy enough to make these gluten-free. Substitute the all-purpose flour with 1 cup white rice flour plus ¾ cup tapioca flour. The texture will be a little grittier than wheat flour dough, but the cookies will still be creamy and irresistible, especially if dipped in chocolate!

Morsels

This recipe is ideal if you have dreams of making vegan cookie dough ice cream at home. Pat the cookie dough into a ½-inch-thick disc between two pieces of waxed paper and freeze until firm. Cut into tiny, bite-size chunks before folding into vanilla or chocolate vegan ice cream.

ACKNOWLEDGMENTS

TERRY WOULD LIKE TO THANK:

John Stavropoulos for swearing the Magical Coconut Bars were better than brownies.

The Audio department for putting up with all of those cookies, week in and week out.

Nerd NYC friends with your helpful stomachs, palates, and hardcore love of cookie dough.

And of course my parents for putting up with a lifetime of me messing up the kitchen.

ISA WOULD LIKE TO THANK:

Justin Field, for putting the chocolate in chip. And doing the dishes.

Marlene Stewart, aka "Mom," for becoming a stage mom later in life.

Portland in general, and Herbivore and Food Fight in particular, for being there for me. (Literally. You are there only for me.)

Fizzle, Avocado and Kirby for being cats.

Jon Hopeless Roberts for teaching me everything I know.

AND THEN, LIKE THE THUNDERCATS, WE FORM ONE GIANT ROBOT AND BOTH THANK:

All who baked cookies and assisted for the photos: Jess DeNoto of Get Sconed, Kimmy Coconut, Michelle Citron, Jawn Dogmatic, Virginia Paine, and Evan "RayRay" McGraw

The crew at Perseus: Katie, Christine, Wendie, Georgia, and Wesley

Our agent, Marc Gerald

And of course, our elite cadre of testers. They gingered the biscotti, black and whited the cookies and oated the meals. And what do they get? An all too brief mention in the back. Thank you guys, for suffering all manners of cookie!!

Amanda Sacco

Ryan Full

Shanell Dawn Williams

Paula Gross

Strummer

Carrie Morse

Luciana Rushing

Monique Martin

Jen Briselli

Teressa Jackson

Thalia C. Palmer

Erica Johnson

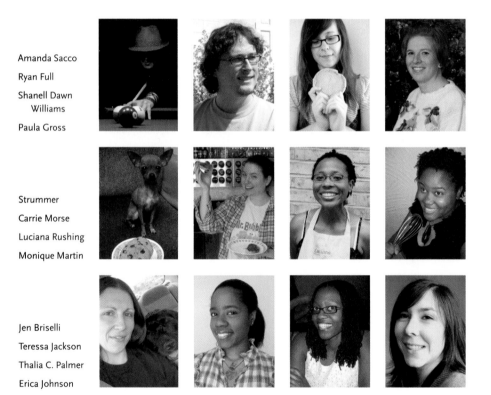

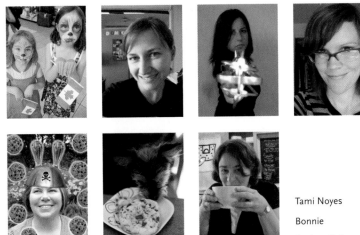
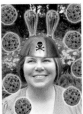
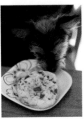
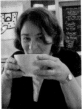

Carla Kelly,
assisted by
Mhairi and
Rhian

Megan McClellan

Rosy Savoia

Rebecca Padrick

Tami Noyes

Bonnie

Raelene Coburn

ABSENT THAT DAY:

Jess DeNoto

Dylan Powell

Bahar Zaker

Kim Carpenter-Lahn

Karyn Casper

Abby Wohl

Megan Duke

Evan Maxwell William McGraw

METRIC CONVERSIONS

THE RECIPES IN THIS BOOK have not been tested with metric measurements, so some variations might occur.
Remember that the weight of dry ingredients varies according to the volume or density factor: 1 cup of flour weighs far less than 1 cup of sugar, and 1 tablespoon doesn't necessarily hold 3 teaspoons.

GENERAL FORMULA FOR METRIC CONVERSION

Ounces to grams	multiply ounces by 28.35
Grams to ounces	multiply ounces by 0.035
Pounds to grams	multiply pounds by 453.5
Pounds to kilograms	multiply pounds by 0.45
Cups to liters	multiply cups by 0.24
Fahrenheit to Celsius	subtract 32 from Fahrenheit temperature,-multiply by 5, divide by 9
Celsius to Fahrenheit	multiply Celsius temperature by 9, divided by 5, add 32

VOLUME (LIQUID) MEASUREMENTS

1 teaspoon = ⅙ fluid ounce = 5 milliliters
1 tablespoon = ½ fluid ounce = 15 milliliters
2 tablespoons = 1 fluid ounce = ⅛ cup,
6 teaspoons = 30 milliliters
¼ cup = 2 fluid ounces = 60 milliliters
⅓ cup = 2 ⅔ fluid ounces = 79 milliliters
½ cup = 4 fluid ounces = 118 milliliters
1 cup = 8 fluid ounces = ½ pint = 250 milliliters
2 cups or 1 pint = 16 fluid ounces = 500 milliliters
4 cups or 1 quart = 32 fluid ounces = 1,000 milliliters
1 gallon = 4 liters

VOLUME (DRY) MEASUREMENTS

¼ teaspoon = 1 milliliter
½ teaspoon = 2 milliliters
¾ teaspoon = 4 milliliters
1 teaspoon = 5 milliliters
1 tablespoon = 15 milliliters
¼ cup = 59 milliliters
⅓ cup = 79 milliliters
½ cup = 118 milliliters
⅔ cup = 158 milliliters
¾ cup = 177 milliliters
1 cup = 225 milliliters
4 cups or 1 quart = 1 liter
½ gallon = 2 liters
1 gallon = 4 liters

WEIGHT (MASS) MEASUREMENTS

1 ounce = 30 grams
2 ounces = 55 grams
3 ounces = 85 grams
4 ounces = ¼ pound = 125 grams
8 ounces = ½ pound = 240 grams
12 ounces = ¾ pound = 375 grams
16 ounces = 1 pound = 454 grams

LINEAR MEASUREMENTS

½ inch = 1 ½ cm
1 inch = 2 ½ cm
6 inches = 15 cm
8 inches = 20 cm
10 inches = 25 cm
12 inches = 30 cm
20 inches = 50 cm

OVEN TEMPERATURE EQUIVALENTS, FAHRENHEIT (F) AND CELSIUS (C)

100°F = 38°C
200°F = 95°C
250°F = 120°C
300°F = 150°C
350°F = 180°C
400°F = 205°C
450°F = 230° C

INDEX